Ketogenic Diet for Beginners

Easy Weight Loss with Plans & Recipes

By Sydney Foster

© 2017

Any advice given in this book is for informational purposes only and is not considered to cure, treat, or prevent any disease. Should you need medical attention, please visit your doctor or an experienced dietician. Always consult your doctor first before starting any type of a diet program.

Free Bonus Content!!

- Free recipes every week
- Free tips on Keto success
- Free meal plans
- Free notification of new books
- And more!

KetoDiet.coach has got you covered!

Visit our website at: http://KetoDiet.coach to sign up for our newsletter free!

Table of Contents

Introduction

Many people have tried to lose weight in one way or another, and people often turn to the ketogenic diet to lose the weight they want successfully. With the wrong diet plan, you may lose the weight and often gain it back right after. The ketogenic diet allows you to lose weight in an effective manner, have more energy in your day to day life, and it will improve your overall health. The best part is that you won't be driven up the wall with hunger pangs when you follow this diet properly. The ketogenic diet focuses on low carbohydrate intake, and then it allows for moderate protein as well a healthy fat. This will keep the fat burning process working even when you sleep. In this book you'll learn why the ketogenic diet works, what you'll need to change to start your keto diet immediately.

Chapter 1: Ketogenic Essentials

Everyone knows that they need energy, and to get energy you need proteins, fats and carbs. Many people have been conditioned to believe that they depend on glucose that comes from carbs to get the energy they need. Only when your glucose that's available starts to become depleted will your body start to break down fat in order to draw energy. The ketogenic diet kick starts this process. A ketogenic diet rarely has any calorie restrictions, and it's a satiating diet because of it. Since this diet keeps you from feeling hungry, your calorie count will naturally fall in line.

Benefits of the Keto Diet

The ketogenic diet, often referred to as the keto diet, has many benefits other than simply turning your body into a fat burning machine.

- **Appetite Control:** The best part about this diet is that you won't be hungry. Your appetite will be regulated and controlled, so you can kiss those hunger pangs goodbye.
- **Mental Clarity:** With a healthy diet, you'll get the nutrients you need in order to increase your mental capabilities.
- **Lowered Inflammation:** Many people won't realize that most of the inflammation they have stems from the food that they eat. With the right diet, you can kiss the inflammation goodbye.
- **Stable Blood Sugar:** Unstable blood sugar levels only leads to health concerns, but with the keto diet you won't have this issue.
- **No Heartburn:** If you are a frequent heart burn sufferer, a keto diet can help with this too.
- **Fat burning & Weight Loss:** This is the most obvious benefit of the keto diet. It makes your body attack the fat to break it down for energy, resulting in the weight loss that you're looking for.

You'll only gain these benefits if you stick with the keto diet. You can't take shortcuts, and you certainly can't have cheat days or breaks. Otherwise you will no longer be in ketosis which is what is causing your fat to burn off.

What Is Ketosis?

You know that ketosis is the state your body has to be in to break down fat, but that doesn't mean you understand it. When the body witches from burning carbs to burning at as its primary source or energy, your body produces ketones. Ketosis is named after these ketones. During ketosis, your blood glucose levels will drop naturally, so there is nothing to worry about. However, it is not recommended that you use a ketogenic diet if you have type 1 diabetes.

The Keto Flu

You should realize that your body will need to adjust to ketosis. Most people experience some discomfort, but it can include constipation, headaches, and diarrhea, lightheadedness, and carb cravings. This is often referred to as the keto flu, but it only affects you when you're just starting your keto lifestyle. This is one of the most common reasons that people claim the diet doesn't work for them. Still, if you stick to it during the transition you'll start to feel better. However, there is no specific time on when these symptoms will go away. Your body is used to burning glucose, not fat. Therefore, it's not going to suddenly learn to go in the opposite direction.

If you're looking to relieve the symptoms while you're sticking with the keto diet, you'll want to add in more fiber such as broccoli and spinach if you're dealing with constipation. If you're dealing with diarrhea you may want to take some more probiotics. For most people, these symptoms won't last more than a few weeks. Some people don't even suffer these symptoms at all. If you feel like this for too long it's because your body is failing to start ketosis. If this is still happening after a few weeks, you need to look at your diet carefully. Chances are that you're still consuming too many carbs or you're under consuming fat. It can be a combination of both. Once you get it sorted out, this should get easier.

You may also experience frequent urination, especially at night. This is usually because your insulin levels are starting to drop. This makes your kidneys begin to flush excess fluid from the body, and this happens to almost everyone in the first few days during ketosis. Once your body adjusts, you'll start evening out again. Your bathroom visits will go back to normal.

Chapter 2: Types of Ketogenic Diets

As your body gets adapted to being in ketosis, you'll feel less hungry. However, there are types of ketogenic diets too, but your body will be able to burn through fat. You should be getting 15-20% protein, 5-15% carbohydrates and 70-75% fats.

Type #1 Standard

This is the standard ketogenic diet, and it's very high in fat and low in carbs. It has moderate protein, and it usually has about twenty percent proteins. It's usually seventy-five percent fat, and usually you're only consuming five percent of carbs. A high protein ketogenic diet can also be included as standard which is thirty-five percent proteins.

Type #2 Cyclical

This is diet consists of ketogenic days that are followed by days that are higher in carbs. This would usually be broken down by five days on the ketogenic diet and two days on a higher-carb diet. Though, some people go a full week with the ketogenic diet and then one higher carb day. This works, but it is known to work slower. It can also cause your weight to vary a little more, especially at first.

Type #3 Targeted

This will give you more freedom to enhance your intake of carbs when you're about to work out. This is better if you're planning to gain more muscle or if you're looking to tone up muscle that you already have. This type of ketogenic diet is not recommended for the average person.

An Important Reminder

It's important to realize that standard and high-protein ketogenic diets are the ones that have been researched and studied. They are the ones that people normally recommend, especially if you're a beginner. The other two methods are only good if you're a bodybuilder or an athlete.

Chapter 3: The Five Steps

Here are the five steps you'll need to introduce your ketogenic diet and clean up your lifestyle. You already know why the keto diet works, but here you'll learn how to maximize your success so that you can lose the weight that you want.

Clean Your Pantry

The first step is to go into your pantry and get rid of the old so that you can bring the new food in. it's not going to help you if you have unhealthy foods tempting you. These temptations are likely to cause failure to any diet, no less one that requires you to be in a state of ketosis. If you don't live alone, this can be a little trickier. If you have to keep items in the house that aren't yours but tempting, try to see if they'll at least keep them out of sight so that you don't feel nearly as tempted.

You'll want to throw out all starches and grains including but not limited to, cereal, pasta, rice, corn, potatoes, quinoa, flour, oats, bagels, wraps, bread, rolls and croissants. Sugary foods and drinks will need to go next because there is no room for refined sugar in the keto diet. Get rid of fountain drinks, milk, fruit juices, pastries, milk chocolate, candy bars, desserts and anything else that fits the bill. Legumes are also bad for your diet, so you'll need to get rid of peas, lentils and beans which are dense with carbs which will skyrocket your glucose levels.

Polyunsaturated fats and oils that have bene processed are also a strict no. get rid of seed oils including canola, soybean, grapeseed, corn oil, safflower and sunflower oil. You'll need to throw out vegetable oils too. Trans fat will need to be eliminated as well, which can be found in both margarine and shortening. If it says hydrogenate or partially hydrogenated, it'll need to go. Keto friendly oils you'll want to replace these with are olive oil, avocado oil and coconut oil.

Fruits can be one of the hardest things to get rid of, but many of them are high in carbs and need cut out. Get rid of mangos, grapes, apples, bananas and dates. Dried fruits such as raisins will need to go too because they're more concentrated and will raise your sugar levels much more quickly in a small serving. Just keep in mind that just because you need to get rid of these foods, doesn't mean that they can't be of use to others. There are many food banks or even online groups that will help you to distribute the food you get rid of to those in need.

Start Shopping

This will be your next step when it comes to committing to your keto diet. After all the food you've thrown out, you'll need to restock. Start with the basics. You'll want to stock up on your spices and herbs, sweeteners which include Erythritol and stevia, lime and lemon juice, water, coffee and tea. You'll also want low carb condiments such as mayonnaise, pesto, sriracha, and mustard. Bone, beef and chicken broth will also be needed. Picked food sand fermented foods can be good to have as well. You'll also want nuts and seeds including pumpkin seeds, chia seed, flaxseed, pine nuts, almonds, pecans, hazelnuts, macadamia nuts and walnuts.

Any type of meat will work for the keto diet, including pork, turkey, game, beef, lamb, chicken and fish. If you can get them, it would be best to stick to grass fed or organic meats. Though, avoid meats that have fat on them and avoid chicken with the skin on it. Wild caught fish and seafood are great, but try to avoid any fish that has been farmed. You can also stock up on eggs. Vegetables may seem like an obvious choice, but there will be some vegetables that you'll need to avoid. You'll have to avoid starchy vegetables, so stick to non-starchy veggies including mushrooms, cucumbers, broccoli, asparagus, lettuce, peppers, tomatoes, onions, garlic, eggplant, olives, zucchini, yellow squash, cauliflower and Brussel sprouts.

There are some fruits that you'll be able to eat such as berries, lemons, limes, and you can also add in avocados. Dairy can be eaten if it's full dairy but you'll need to avoid sweetened yogurt, skim milk and regular whole milk. Butter, sour cream, heavy whipping cream, cheese, cream cheese and unsweetened yogurt go into your keto diet nicely, though. You can also use coconut milk and almond milk if it's unsweetened.

When it comes to oils, you already know that you can use avocado oil and olive oil. You can also use real butter, lard and even bacon fat. If you aren't used to using avocado oil, keep in mind that it has a high smoke point which makes it perfect for searing meats or even using in a wok. Just avoid an oil that is labeled 'blend' because it'll have a small amount of healthy oil but large amounts of unhealthy oils to make it a cheaper option.

Stock Your Kitchen

When you're preparing recipes, it's going to be easier if you have the right tools. With the right tools, cooking becomes faster and simpler, meaning less work and less stress for you. Here are a few things you'll need in order to stock your kitchen.

- **Food Scale:** If you're trying to hit a certain goal, you'll want to have a food scale on hand. You can usually get a food scale online for as little as ten dollars.
- **Electric Hand Mixer:** Some recipes require you to beat egg whites until you get stiff peaks, and doing this by hand will be difficult. An electric hand mixer can be bought for as little as ten dollars, and it'll save you a lot of trouble.
- **Food Processor:** This will help you to blend food into a sauce or shake, and a blender just won't work. It doesn't have the power to blend certain tough vegetables.
- **Cast Iron Pans:** This is a preference, but it can be a healthier option to cook in since it has no chemical treatment of any kind. They also retain heat well, and they can be used in both the oven and on the stove. Just wash them with a scrub sponge without soap, dry them off and then coat in cooking oil to clean, which makes cleaning up a brief.
- **Knife Sharpening Stone:** Most food preparation involves cutting, which will quickly become a pain if you have doll knives. You should aim to sharpen your knives on a weekly basis if you want them to stay sharp.
- **Spiralizer:** This will help you to make vegetables into noodles, which can help you to get a keto friendly version of any of your favorite pasta dishes. It comes in handy once you've gotten rid of the starches that will set your weight loss goals back.

Meal Planning

Meal planning won't always be necessary, but it's good to start off with if you want to ensure the success of your diet. If you know when you're going to eat, what you're going to eat and even prep it at certain times, then you're more likely to stick to the diet that you've chosen. Just commit to meal planning and meal preparation for a little while and it'll help you to stay focused, and you may even find that you get the hang of it and like doing it. After all, many people believe that it helps to make their life a little easier.

You'll find meal plans for every part of your day in this book. Having a meal plan gives you direction on where to go with your diet, making it less daunting. It also gives you goals that you can meet. Sticking to your meal plan is an accomplishment, and it's something you'll need to strive for. It also gives you something to look forward to when you know what you're going to eat. You can use the meal plan in this book as many times as you like, but keep in mind that you can customize them as well.

There are also recipes in this book that you can use to help swap out recipes in the meal plans that have been provided. Remember that caloric goals don't have to be exact. You can usually go one or two hundred calories in either direction, or you'll still be fine. You can even use an online keto calculator when you're creating a meal plan of your own. If you're looking to get about an extra hundred calories, then just use another tablespoon of olive oil or butter. When creating your email plan, you'll need to look for the right ingredients when shopping too. Always look at your nutritional labels so that you know everything that you're putting in your body.

Add in Exercise

You'll still need to add in some exercise with your ketogenic diet if you want the pounds to melt away. If you don't exercise right now, you'll want to start off slow. Make sure to take short walks, slow jogs, or just exercise lightly for fifteen minutes a day. If you do already go to the gym, then add a little more weight, add some time to your exercise or do a little more cardio. Just try to do a little more than what you're doing now, and it'll help you to become a little healthier. It can even be helpful if you decide to take a class or start to play a sport. With the keto diet and light exercise, both of your health and your energy levels should improve.

Chapter 4: Two Week Meal Plan

Here's a two week meal plan to start with, but remember that you can customize it as necessary. Though, it's best to stick to this meal plan when you're just starting off to ensure that you have the right balance to get over the keto flu as quickly as possible. This meal plan is based on twenty net carbs a day, and the snacks you choose will depend on how many net carbs are left.

Week #1

Sunday

Breakfast: Mocha Chia Pudding

Net Carbs: 2.25 Grams

Lunch: Brussels Salad

Net Carbs: 5 Grams

Dinner: Pumpkin Curry

Net Carbs: 7 Grams

Snack Allowance: 5.75

Monday

Breakfast: Green Smoothie

Net Carbs: 6 Grams

Lunch: Pizza Bread

Net Carbs: 1.9 Grams

Dinner: Chicken & Broccoli Alfredo

Net Carbs: 1 Gram

Snack Allowance: 11.1 Grams

Tuesday

Breakfast: Strawberry & Chia Breakfast

Net Carbs: 7.5 Grams

Lunch: Pesto Gnocchi

Net Carbs: 7 Grams

Dinner: Vegetable Fried Beef

Net Carbs: 3 Grams

Snack Allowance: 2.5

Wednesday

Breakfast: Keto French Toast

Net Carbs: 3.3 Grams

Lunch: Cheesy Baked Zoodles

Net Carbs: 6 Grams

Dinner: Leek & Bacon Frittata

Net Carbs: 3 Grams

Snack Allowance: 7.7 Grams

Thursday

Breakfast: Baked Brie with Pecans

Net Carbs: 0.43 Grams

Lunch: Salmon Poke Bowl

Net Carbs: 8.5 Grams

Dinner: Spiced Lobster Salad

Net Carbs: 2 Grams

Snack Allowance: 9.07

Friday

Breakfast: Breakfast Mug Muffin

Net Carbs: 3.4 Grams

Lunch: Egg Drop Soup

Net Carbs: 2.9 Grams

Dinner: Skillet Salmon

Net Carbs: 1 Gram

Side Dish: Creamy Spinach

Net Carbs: 1 Gram

Snack Allowance: 11.7 Grams

Saturday

Breakfast: Chia & Pumpkin Muffins

Net Carbs: 3 Grams

Lunch: Ricotta & Lemon Zoodles

Net Carbs: 4 Grams

Dinner: Coconut Lime Steak

Net Carbs: 3 Grams

Side Dish: Easy Brussel Sprouts

Net Carbs: 6.8 Grams

Snack Allowance: 3.2 Grams

Week #2

Sunday

Breakfast: Pumpkin Pancakes

Net Carbs: 5 Grams

Lunch: Blue Cheese Zoodles

Net Carbs: 5 Grams

Dinner: Wrapped Tilapia

Net Carbs: 2 Grams

Side Dish: Ranch Broccoli Bites

Net Carbs: 4 Grams

Snack Allowance: 4 Grams

Monday

Breakfast: Artichoke & Bacon Omelet

Net Carbs: 3 Grams

Lunch: Greek Salad

Net Carbs: 8 Grams

Dinner: Coffee Tuna Steak

Net Carbs: 2 Grams

Side Dish: Kale Slaw

Net Carbs: 3.5 Grams

Snack Allowance: 3.5 Grams

Tuesday

Breakfast: Egg Pesto Muffins

Net Carbs: 1.2 Grams

Lunch: Spinach Tabbouleh

Net Carbs: 5.4 Grams

Dinner: Cheesy Italian Meatballs

Net Carbs: 4 Grams

Side Dish: Roasted Broccoli

Net Carbs: 6.9 Grams

Snack Allowance: 2.5 Grams

Wednesday

Breakfast: Easy Breakfast Bake

Net Carbs: 3 Grams

Lunch: Vietnamese Pho

Net Carbs: 6.5 Grams

Dinner: Beef Roll Ups

Net Carbs: 1 Gram

Side Dish: Southern Green Beans

Net Carbs: 4 Grams

Snack Allowance: 5.5 Grams

Thursday

Breakfast: Rosemary Quiche

Net Carbs: 1 Grams

Lunch: Duck Ramen

Net Carbs: 7.1 Grams

Dinner: Walnut Pork Chops

Net Carbs: 1 Gram

Side Dish: Rosti

Net Carbs: 3 Grams

Snack Allowance: 7.9 Grams

Friday

Breakfast: Cheese & Chive Scones

Net Carbs: 1.3 Grams

Lunch: Tricolore Salad

Net Carbs: 8.6 Grams

Dinner: Cajun Snow Crab

Net Carbs: 3 Grams

Side Dish: Crisp Zucchini

Net Carbs: 1 Gram

Snack Allowance: 6.1 Grams

Saturday

Breakfast: Breakfast Hash

Net Carbs: 6.6 Grams

Lunch: Butternut & Turkey Soup

Net Carbs: 3.25 Grams

Dinner: Easy Black Pepper Chicken

Net Carbs: 4 Grams

Side Dish: Asparagus & Walnuts

Net Carbs: 2 Grams

Snack Allowance: 4.15 Grams

Chapter 5: Breakfast Recipes

In this chapter you'll find all the breakfast recipes you need for your meal plan, as well as a few others.

Mocha Chia Pudding

Time: 35 Minutes

Calories: 257

Fat: 20.25

Net Carbs: 2.25

Fiber: 11.5

Protein: 7 Grams

Ingredients:

- 2 Tablespoons Herbal Coffee
- 1/3 Cup Coconut Cream, Undiluted
- 2 Tablespoons Cacao Nibs
- 1 Tablespoon Vanilla Extract, Pure
- 1 Tablespoon Sweetener
- 1/3 Cup Chia Seeds, Dry

Directions:

1. Start by brewing a strong herbal coffee by taking two tablespoons of herbal blend with two cups of water, and then let it seep for fifteen minute. The liquid should be reduced to about a cup. Keep the rest for later.
2. Blend in your coconut cream and herbal coffee, and then add in your sweetener such as swerve. Next, you'll want to add in your vanilla extract.
3. Add your chia seeds and cacao nibs, stirring together.
4. Place in a container and chill for at least a half hour before serving.

Keto Muffins

Yield: 10

Serving Size: 1 Muffin

Calories: 128

Fat: 10 Grams

Net Carbs: 2.5 Grams

Fiber: 0.75 Grams

Protein: 6.6 Grams

Time: 40 Minutes

Ingredients:

- 2 Tablespoons Drippings (Steak or Bacon)
- ½ Cup Almond Flour
- ½ Cup Roasted Tomatillo Salsa
- 4 Eggs, Medium
- 1 Ounce Beef Jerky Manchaca

Directions:

1. Start by heating your oven to 350.
2. Take a nonstick pan, and melt the fat of your choice, adding in your machaca. Stir and cook for about three minutes until it's softened as well as fragrant. You'll need to let it cool for five minutes.
3. Take a food processor and blend your machaca, almond flour, eggs and tomatillo salsa. Blend on low for about thirty seconds, and then pour into muffin tins.
4. Bake at 30 for about a half hour. A toothpick should be able to come out clean when inserted in the middle.

Cheese & Chive Scones

Serves: 15

Calories: 127

Fat: 2.3 Grams

Protein: 5.7 Grams

Fiber: 2.2 Grams

Net Carbs: 1.3 Grams

Time: 25 Minutes

Ingredients:

- 1 ½ Cups Almond Flour
- 2 Eggs, Medium
- 1 Teaspoon Baking Powder
- ¼ Cup Coconut Flour
- ¼ Cup Flax Seeds
- 4 Slices Bacon
- 2-3 Tablespoons Chives, Chopped
- 1.8 Ounces Cheddar, Grated
- ½ Teaspoon Black Pepper
- ¼ Teaspoon Sea Salt, Fine
- 3 Tablespoons Almond Milk, Unsweetened

Directions:

1. Start by heating you oven to 375, and then blend your flaxseeds until ground in a blender.
2. Combine your flax, almonds, baking powder, coconut flour, cheese, chives, salt and pepper in a bowl. Mix it well.
3. Chop your bacon, and then fry for three to four minutes. Allow your bacon to cool.
4. Crack your eggs in a cup, whisking before adding your almond milk. Mix again.
5. Add your wet ingredients to your dry ingredients, forming a dough. Stir this through your bacon.
6. Roll your dough between paper, and then cut into cookie shapes.

7. Bake for fifteen minutes, and sprinkle cheese over them after ten minutes.

Strawberry & Chia Breakfast

Serves: 4

Calories: 230

Fiber: 4 Grams

Protein: 8.7 Grams

Fat: 17.9 Grams

Net Carbs: 7.5 Grams

Time: 40 Minutes

Ingredients:

Chia Layer:

- ¼ Teaspoon Cinnamon
- 1 Cup Coconut Milk
- ¼ Teaspoon Ground Ginger
- 4 Tablespoons Chia Seeds

Strawberry Layer:

- 2 Tablespoons Water
- 1 Cup Strawberries

Yogurt & Strawberry Layer:

- 4 Strawberries, Large & Sliced
- 1 Cup Yogurt, Full Fat

Directions:

1. Slice your strawberries, and then place your sliced strawberries in two tablespoons of water. Bring to a simmer, and cook for a few minutes until softened.
2. Break them apart with a spatula. Add in a few drops of stevia if desired.
3. Mix the chia seeds, ginger powder, coconut milk, and cinnamon together.
4. Set this to the side, letting it soak for twenty to thirty minutes.
5. Divide your chia mixture between four jars.
6. Add your cooked strawberries to make another layer.

7. Add your full fat yogurt as your next layer.
8. Serve cooled.

Chocolate & Mint Smoothie

Serves: 1

Calories: 401

Fiber: 7.8 Grams

Protein: 5 Grams

Fat: 40.3 Grams

Net Carbs: 6.5 Grams

Time: 5 Minutes

Ingredients:

- 1 Cup Almond Milk, Unsweetened
- ¼ Cup Coconut Milk
- 1 Tablespoon Cocoa Powder, Unsweetened
- ½ Avocado, Medium
- 3 Ice Cubes
- 4-6 Mint Leaves
- 1 Tablespoon MCT Oil
- 2 Tablespoons Liquid Sweetener

Directions:

1. Blend everything until smooth.

Macha & Almond Smoothie

Serves: 1

Calories: 500

Protein: 14.6 Grams

Fiber: 4.7 Grams

Fat: 43.8 Grams

Net Carbs: 6.2 Grams

Time: 5 Minutes

Ingredients:

- ¾ Cup Almond Milk, Unsweetened
- 1 Tablespoon Almond Butter
- ¼ Cup Coconut Milk, Unsweetened
- 2 Tablespoons Macha Powder
- 1 Tablespoon Collagen Powder
- 1 Tablespoon Coconut Oil
- ½ Teaspoon Ground Cinnamon

Directions:

1. Blend well until smooth. Serve chilled.

Baked Brie with Pecans

Serves: 1

Calories: 183

Fat: 16.5 Grams

Net Carbs: 0.43 Grams

Fiber: 1 Gram

Protein: 8.42 Grams

Time: 20 Minutes

Ingredients:

- 1/8 Teaspoon Black Pepper
- 6 Pecan Halves (1/3 Ounce)
- 1 Ounce Brie Cheese, Full Fat
- 1 Slice Prosciutto (1/2 Ounce)

Directions:

1. Start by heating your oven to 350, and then use a muffin tin and prepare it.
2. Fold your prosciutto slice in half, and then place it in your muffin tin.
3. Chop your brie into cubes, but leave the white skin on. Place it in your prosciutto lined cup.
4. Stick the pecan halves in the brie.

5. Bake for about twelve minutes. Your prosciutto should cook and your brie should melt.
6. Let it cool before eating.

Buttered Green Eggs

Serves: 2

Calories: 311

Fat: 27.5 Grams

Net Carbs: 2.5 Grams

Fiber: 1 Gram

Protein: 12.8 Grams

Time: 20 Minutes

Ingredients:

- 2 Tablespoons Butter, Pastured
- 1 Tablespoon Coconut oil
- ½ Cup Cilantro, Fresh & Chopped
- ½ Cup Parsley, Fresh & Chopped
- 4 Medium Eggs
- 1 Teaspoon Thyme Leaves, Fresh
- 2 Garlic Cloves, Peeled & Chopped Fine
- ¼ Teaspoon Ground Cayenne
- ¼ Teaspoon Ground Cumin
- ½ Teaspoon Sea Salt, Fine

Directions:

1. Melt your butter and coconut oil for a minute, and then add in your chopped garlic. Cook for about three minutes on low. Your garlic should start to brown.
2. Add in your thyme, browning for thirty seconds. Be careful not to let either burn.
3. Add in your parsley and cilantro, cooking on medium for about three minutes. You want these to become slightly crisp.
4. Add in your eggs, and try not to break the yolk.
5. Cover the pan, and then reduce to low.
6. Cook for four to six minutes, and the yolks should still be soft.
7. Serve immediately.

Green Smoothie

Serves: 1

Calories: 468

Fiber: 5.4 Grams

Protein: 4.2 Grams

Fat: 48.2 Grams

Net Carbs: 6 Grams

Time: 5 Minutes

Ingredients:

- ½ Avocado, Medium
- ½ Cup Coconut Milk, Unsweetened
- ½ Cup Spinach, Fresh
- ½-3/4 Cup Water + 2-3 Ice Cubes
- 1 Teaspoon Vanilla Extract, Pure
- 2 Tablespoons Swerve
- 1 Teaspoon Matcha Powder
- 1 Tablespoon Coconut Oil

Directions:

1. Halve your avocado, peel and remove the seed.
2. Place all ingredients in a blender, and blend until smooth.
3. Add more ice if you want to thicken.

Cinnamon Smoothie

Serves: 1

Calories: 467

Fiber: 3.5 Grams

Protein: 23.6 Grams

Fat: 40.3 Grams

Net Carbs: 4.7 Grams

Time: 5 Minutes

Ingredients:

- ½ Cup Water
- 2 Ice Cubes
- 1 Tablespoon Coconut Oil
- ½ Cup Coconut Milk
- 1 Tablespoon Chia Seeds, Ground
- ½-1 Teaspoon Cinnamon
- ¼ Cup Vanilla Whey Powder

Directions:

1. Blend everything together and serve immediately.

Breakfast Mug Muffin

Serves: 2

Calories: 390

Fiber: 6.7 Grams

Protein: 19.7 Grams

Fat: 31.2 Grams

Net Carbs: 3.4 Grams

Time: 10 Minutes

Ingredients:

- ¼ Cup Flax meal
- ¼ Cup almond Flour
- ¼ Teaspoon Baking Soda
- 1 Egg, Large
- 2 Tablespoons Water
- ½ Teaspoon Sea Salt, Fine
- 2 Tablespoons Coconut Milk, Unsweetened
- 3 Slices Bacon, Cooked & Crumbled
- 3 Tablespoons Spinach, Cooked & Drained
- 1.8 Ounces Feta Cheese, Crumbled

Directions:

1. Start by combining all dry ingredients in a bowl.
2. Add your milk, egg, and water to your mix, mixing well.
3. Add in your bacon, cheese and spinach, mixing well.
4. Microwave for sixty to ninety seconds, and then let it sit for five minutes before enjoying.

Keto French Toast

Serves: 4

Calories: 546

Fiber: 0.9 Grams

Protein: 32.7 Grams

Fat: 47.5 Grams

Net Carbs: 3.3 Grams

Time: 10 Minutes

Ingredients:

- 1 Tablespoon Heavy Whipping Cream
- 1 Teaspoon Cinnamon + Extra for Dusting
- ½ Teaspoon Sea Salt, Fine
- 1/8 Teaspoon Ground Nutmeg
- 2 Tablespoons Coconut Oil
- 1 Tablespoon Swerve
- 1 Tablespoon Water
- 2 Eggs, Large
- 8 Slices Keto Bread, Sliced ½ Inch Thick

Directions:

1. Place your swerve, cinnamon, nutmeg, water, salt, cream and eggs together. Whisk with a fork.
2. Grease a pan with ghee, and place it over medium-high heat. Dip your bread into it, and then place in a hot pan.
3. Cook on each side for thirty to forty seconds until browned lightly.
4. Place two slices per serving on a plate, and then dust with cinnamon.

Keto Fiber Cereal

Serves: 4

Calories: 254

Fat: 15.5 Grams

Net Carbs: 1.5

Fiber: 15.6 Grams

Protein: 9.2 Grams

Time: 1 Hour 10 Minutes

Ingredients:

- ½ Cup Chia Seeds
- 1 Cup Water
- 2 Tablespoons Coconut Oil, Melted
- 1 Tablespoon Psyllium Powder
- 4 Tablespoons Hemp Hearts
- 2 Tablespoons Raw Cacao Nibs
- 1 Tablespoon Sweetener (Such as Swerve)
- 1 Tablespoon Vanilla Extract, Pure

Directions:

1. Start by heating your oven to 300.
2. Combine your chia seeds and water in a bowl, and set it aside for about five minutes.
3. Add the rest of your ingredients except your cacao nibs into the bowl.
4. Mix all ingredients together.
5. Add in your cacao nibs, and then stir them into the dough.
6. Roll out, and then place with the shiny side up on parchment paper. Flatten the dough with your fingertips.
7. Cover, and then roll out to ¼ inch thickness. It should make about eighteen inches.
8. Peel the top paper from your dough.
9. Bake on 15 minutes until dry, and then remove from the oven. Flip, and then bake for another 15-25 minutes.

10. Remove from the oven and allow to cool. Cut into inch squares, and then store for about three days. Serve with almond or coconut milk.

Strawberry & Black Currant Smoothie

Serves: 1

Calories: 228

Fiber: 9.4 Grams

Protein: 5.1 Grams

Fat: 17.3 Grams

Net Carbs: 8.7 Grams

Time: 5 Minutes

Ingredients:

- ¼ Cup Strawberries, Fresh or Frozen
- ¼ Cup Coconut Milk
- ½ Cup Black Currants, Fresh or Frozen
- ½ Cup Water
- 2 Tablespoons Chia Seeds, Powdered
- ½ Vanilla Bean

Directions:

1. Blend everything together until smooth and then serve immediately.

Chia & Pumpkin Muffins

Serves: 12

Calories: 211

Fiber: 3. Grams

Fat: 18.5 Grams

Protein: 7.3 Grams

Net Carbs: 3 Grams

Time: 45 Minutes

Ingredients:

- 1 ½ Cups Almond Flour
- 1 Tablespoons Pumpkin Pie Spice Mix
- 1 Tablespoons Baking Powder
- ¼ Cup Chia Seeds, Ground
- 6 Tablespoons Pumpkin Seeds
- ¼ Cup Swerve, Powdered
- 20-30 Drops Liquid Stevia
- ½ Cup Butter
- 6 Eggs, Large & Separated
- 1 Cup Pumpkin Puree
- Melted Ghee for Greasing

Directions:

1. Start by heating your oven to 350.
2. Combine all dry ingredients together besides your pumpkin seeds, combining well.
3. Separate your egg yolks and egg whites together. Beat the egg whites together, creating soft peaks.
4. Place your egg yolks, pumpkin puree, melted butter and stevia together.
5. Add your dry mix a tablespoon at a time, and then add a quarter of your egg whites together, mixing gently. Add the remaining by folding it in slowly.
6. Line your muffin trays with paper cups, and then grease them.
7. Spoon your batter into the paper cups.

8. Bake for five minutes, and then sprinkle the pumpkin seeds on top.
9. Bake for another thirty minutes. The tops should be golden brown. These will keep four to five days.

Complete Keto Breakfast

Serves: 2

Calories: 313

Fat: 26 Grams

Net Carbs: 2.5

Fiber: 6 Grams

Protein: 13 Grams

Time: 15 Minutes

Ingredients:

- 4 Strips Bacon, Uncured
- 2 Large Eggs
- ¼ Teaspoon Sea Salt, Fine
- 1 Large Avocado, Peeled & Sliced

Directions:

1. Put your avocado and bacon into a frying pan over medium heat, and then flip after three minutes.
2. Remove from the pan, and then leave the dripping sin it. Cook your eggs like you like, and then enjoy.

Breakfast Frittata

Serves: 4

Calories: 313

Fat: 30 Grams

Net Carbs: 2.4

Fiber: 3.25

Protein: 9 Grams

Time: 15 Minutes

Ingredients:

- 4 Eggs, Medium
- 10 Olives, Pitted
- 2 Ounces Brie Cheese, Full Fat
- 2 Tablespoons Olive Oil
- 2 Tablespoons Butter
- ½ Teaspoon Sea Salt, Fine
- 1 Avocado, Medium
- 1 Teaspoon Herbes de Provence

Directions:

1. Take a large bowl and blend your eggs, herbes de Provence, olives, salt and oil together until frothy.
2. Peel and slice your avocado, making thick slices.
3. Melt your butter in a saucepan, and then add in your avocado. Fry in butter until golden on both sides, and then set it aside.
4. Coo your eggs as desired, and then slice your brie, and then place it on your egg mixture.
5. Cover the skillet and cook for three minutes. It should become golden brown, and use a plate to flip and cook your frittata for about two more minutes. Top with avocado before serving.

Salmon & Cheese Mug Muffin

Serves: 2

Calories: 374

Fiber: 6.5 Grams

Protein: 17.2 Grams

Fat: 32.3 Grams

Net Carbs: 3 Grams

Time: 10 Minutes

Ingredients:

- ¼ Cup Almond Flour
- ¼ Teaspoon Baking Soda
- 2 Tablespoons Water
- 1 Egg, Large
- 2 Tablespoons Coconut Milk, Unsweetened
- ¼ Teaspoon Sea Salt, Fine
- ¼ Teaspoon Baking Soda
- ¼ Cup Flax meal
- 2 Tablespoons Water
- 2.1 Ounces Smoked Salmon
- 2 Tablespoons Chives, Fresh & Chopped
- 2.1 Ounces Cream Cheese, Full Fat

Directions:

1. Combine all dry ingredients together.
2. Add your water, milk and egg together, mixing well.
3. Slice your smoked salmon and chop your chives, adding it to the mixture.
4. Split into two mugs.
5. Microwave for sixty to ninety seconds, and then top with your cream cheese.

Pumpkin Pancakes

Serves: 2

Calories: 443

Fat: 35 Grams

Net Carbs: 5 Grams

Fiber: 7 Grams

Protein: 21 Grams

Time: 35 Minutes

Ingredients:

- 2 Ounces Ground Flax Seeds
- 2 Ounces Hazelnut Flour
- 1 Ounce Egg White Protein
- 1 Teaspoon Baking Powder, Aluminum Free
- 1 Tablespoons Chai Masala Mix
- 1 Teaspoon Vanilla Extract, Pure
- 3 Eggs, Medium
- 4-5 Drops Liquid Sweetener
- Coconut Oil to Fry
- 1 Cup Coconut Cream
- ½ Cup Pumpkin Puree

Directions:

1. Mix all of your wet ingredient into a bowl until frothy.
2. Mix both your flours, masala mix, sweetener, baking powder and salt together.
3. Add your dry and wet ingredients together, whisking well.
4. Add ¼ cup of water if it's too dry, and then heat your oil in a pan.
5. Pour in enough for a pancake, cooking like normal. It'll tea about two to three minutes on each side.
6. Serve immediately. You may also want to serve with coconut cream on top.

Breakfast Hash

Serves: 1

Calories: 423

Fat: 35.5 Grams

Net Carbs: 6.6 Grams

Fiber: 2.5 Grams

Protein: 17.4 Grams

Time: 25 Minutes

Ingredients:

- 1 Tablespoon Coconut Oil
- 1 Egg, Large
- ¼ Teaspoon Sea Salt, Fine
- 1 Tablespoon Chives, Freshly Chopped
- ½ White Onion, Small
- 2 Slices Bacon
- 1 Zucchini, Medium

Directions:

1. Start by chopping your onion.
2. Cook your onion and bacon until lightly browned.
3. Dice your zucchini, and then add to the pan. Cook for another ten to fifteen minutes, and then remove from heat.
4. Add in your chopped parsley.
5. Fry your egg as desired and place it on top your hash before serving.

Fisherman's Eggs

Serves: 1

Calories: 315

Protein: 28 Grams

Fat: 20.63 Grams

Fiber: 1.3 Grams

Net Carbs: 3.5 Grams

Time: 15 Minutes

Ingredients:

- 2 Eggs, Medium
- 56 Grams Sardines in Olive Oil
- ½ Cap Arugula
- 2 ½ Tablespoons Marinated Artichoke Hearts
- ¼ Teaspoon Sea Salt, Fine
- ¼ Teaspoon Black Pepper

Directions:

1. Start by heating your oven to 375.
2. Put your sardines in the bottom of an oven proof stoneware dish.
3. Break your eggs on top, and then add in your artichokes and arugula.
4. Add in your salt and pepper, and then bake at 375 for ten minutes.
5. Serve immediately.

Egg Pesto Muffins

Serves: 10

Calories: 125

Fiber: 0.7 Grams

Fat: 10.2 Grams

Protein: 6.9 Grams

Net Carbs: 1.2 Grams

Time: 30 Minutes

Ingredients:

- 4.4 Ounces Goat Cheese
- 6 Eggs, Large
- Salt & Pepper to Taste
- ½ Cup Olives, Pitted
- ¼ Cup Sun Dried Tomatoes, Chopped
- 3 Tablespoons Pesto
- 2/3 Cup Frozen Spinach, Thawed & Drained

Directions:

1. Start by heating your oven to 350, and then squeeze any water from your spinach. Deseed olives, and then slice them. Chop your sundried tomatoes, and crack your eggs in a bowl.
2. Add pesto to the eggs, and season with your salt and pepper. Make sure to mix well.
3. Crumble your goat cheese into your muffin tins. Add in spinach, olives and sun dried tomatoes.
4. Pour your egg and pesto mix on top, and bake for twenty to twenty-five minutes.
5. It will last in the fridge for five days.

Nut Medley Granola

Serves: 8

Calories: 391

Fat: 38 Grams

Protein: 10 Grams

Fiber: 6 Grams

Net Carbs: 4 Grams

Time: 1 Hour

Ingredients:

- 2 Cups Coconut, Shredded & Unsweetened
- 1 Cup Sunflower Seeds, Raw
- 1 Cup Almonds, Sliced
- 10 Drops Liquid Stevia
- ½ Cup Walnuts
- ½ Cup Coconut Oil, Melted
- ½ Cup Pumpkin Seeds, Raw
- 1 Teaspoon Ground Cinnamon
- ½ Teaspoon Ground Nutmeg

Directions:

1. Start by heating your oven to 250, and then line two baking sheets using parchment paper before setting them aside.
2. Toss the almonds, shredded coconut, pumpkin seeds, sunflower seeds, and walnuts together, mixing well.
3. Stir together your coconut oil, cinnamon, stevia and nutmeg until blended well.
4. Pour in your coconut oil mixture into your nut mixture, and then blend well using your hands.
5. Transfer your granola to a baking sheet, spreading evenly.
6. Bake your granola, stirring about every ten to fifteen minutes. It should turn golden brown, which should take about an hour.
7. Transfer to a large bowl, and break up into large pieces.
8. Store in an airtight container. You can freeze it up to a month.

Scrambled Pesto Eggs

Serves: 1

Calories: 467

Fiber: 0.7 Grams

Protein: 20.4 Grams

Fat: 41.5 Grams

Net Carbs: 2.6 Grams

Time: 10 Minutes

Ingredients:

- 3 Eggs, Large
- 1 Tablespoon Pesto
- 1 Tablespoon Butter
- 2 Tablespoons Creamed Coconut Milk
- Salt & Pepper to Taste

Directions:

1. Crack your eggs into a bowl, and then add your salt and pepper. Beat them together, and then pour into a pan.
2. Add in your butter, turning the heat on.
3. Stir constantly, and add the pesto mixture.
4. Take off heat and add in your creamed coconut.
5. Keep cooking until done as desired, and then serve warm.

Artichoke & Bacon Omelet

Serves: 4

Calories: 435

Fat: 39 Grams

Fiber: 2 Grams

Protein: 17 Grams

Net Carbs: 3 Grams

Time: 10 Minutes

Ingredients:

- 6 Eggs, Medium & Beaten
- 1 Tablespoon Olive Oil
- ½ Cup Artichoke Hearts, Chopped
- ¼ Cup Onion, Chopped
- 8 Bacon Slices, Chopped & Cooked
- 2 Tablespoons Heavy Whipping Cream
- ½ Teaspoon Sea Salt, Fine
- ¼ Teaspoon Black Pepper

Directions:

1. Whisk your eggs, heavy cream and bacon together until blended well.
2. Place a skillet over medium-high heat, adding in your olive oil.
3. Sauté your onion for about three minutes until they're tender.
4. Pour your egg mixture in the skillet, and then cook for one minute.
5. Cook your omelet, lifting your edges with a spatula, lifting so that the uncooked egg can flow underneath. Cook for another two minutes.
6. Add in your artichoke hearts before flipping your omelet. Cook for about four more minutes, and then flip again.
7. Remove from heat, and then cut to serve.

Mexican Breakfast Casserole

Serves: 6

Calories: 423

Fiber: 1.7 Grams

Protein: 26.5 Grams

Fat: 31.8 Grams

Net Carbs: 5.5 Grams

Time: 1 Hour

Ingredients:

- 1 lb Bacon, Thick Cut
- 2 Tablespoons Bacon Grease, Reserved
- ½ Cup Cheddar Cheese, Shredded
- ½ Teaspoon Black Pepper
- 1 Teaspoon Garlic Powder
- 1 Teaspoon Sea Salt, Fine
- 12 Eggs, Large
- 1/3 Cup Whole Milk
- 3 Cups Spinach
- 1 Red Onion, Large & Sliced Thin
- 1 Turnip, Small & Diced

Directions:

1. Start by heating your oven to 400.
2. Your bacon needs cut in two inch pieces, and then line a baking sheet with parchment paper. Bake for fifteen minutes, and then bake until crisp.
3. Use your reserved bacon grease in a pan, heating it and cooing the turnip and onion until soft. This should take about five to seven minutes.
4. Use a 9x13 inch pan, and add in your turnip and onion. Top with spinach.
5. Whisk the milk, spices and eggs together, pouring it over your spinach.
6. Sprinkle your cheese on top, and then arrange the bacon on top.
7. Bake for twenty to twenty-five minutes.
8. It'll store in the fridge for five days, but serve warm.

Easy Breakfast Bake

Serves: 8

Calories: 303

Fat: 24 Grams

Protein: 17 Grams

Fiber: 1 Gram

Net Carbs: 3 Grams

Time: 1 Hour

Ingredients:

- 1 Tablespoon Olive Oil + Extra for Greasing
- 8 Large Eggs
- 1 lb Sausage
- 2 Cups Spaghetti Squash, Cooked
- ½ Teaspoon Sea Salt, Fine
- ¼ Teaspoon Ground Black Pepper
- 1 Tablespoon Oregano, Fresh & Chopped
- ½ Cup Cheddar Cheese, Shredded

Directions:

1. Heat your oven to 375, and grease a 9x13 inch dish with olive oil before setting it aside.
2. Add your olive oil to a skillet over medium-high heat.
3. Brown your sausage until cooked, which should take about five minutes.
4. Whisk together your eggs, squash, and oregano in a bowl. Season with salt and pepper.
5. Add your cooked sausage to your egg mix, and then stir until combined. Pour into your casserole.
6. Sprinkle your cheese on top, and cover with aluminum foil loosely.
7. Bake for a half hour, and then remove your foil baking for another fifteen minutes.
8. Let cool before serving.

Cinnamon & Pecan Porridge

Serves: 2

Calories: 580

Protein: 13.8 Grams

Fat: 51.7 Grams

Fiber: 10 Grams

Net Carbs: 5.2 Grams

Time: 20 Minutes

Ingredients:

- ¼ Cup Coconut Milk
- ¾ Cup Almond Milk, Unsweetened
- 1 Tablespoon Coconut Oil
- ¼ Cup Almond Butter
- 2 Tablespoons Chia Seeds, Whole
- 2 Tablespoons Hemp Seeds
- ¼ Cup Chopped Pecans
- ¼ Cup Toasted Coconut, Unsweetened
- ½ Teaspoon Cinnamon
- 4-10 Drops Liquid Sweetener

Directions:

1. Mix your coconut milk, almond milk, coconut oil and almond butter. Simmer over medium heat, and then take off heat once hot.
2. Add in your chopped pecans, hemp seeds, toasted coconut and chia seeds. Reserve some of your toasted coconut for topping.
3. Add in your cinnamon and stevia, letting it sit for five to ten minutes.
4. Serve hot or cold depending on preference.

Rosemary Quiche

Serves: 6

Calories: 184

Total Fat: 14 Grams

Protein: 12 Grams

Fiber: 1 Grams

Net Carbs: 1 Gram

Time: 30 Minutes

Ingredients:

- 1 Teaspoon Olive Oil, Rosemary Infused
- 6 Eggs, Large
- ½ Cup Heavy Whipping Cream
- 7 Ounces Ham, Cubed
- 2 Tablespoon Cream Cheese, Room Temperature
- 1 Teaspoon Rosemary, Fresh & Chopped
- 1 Teaspoon Sea Salt, Fine

Directions:

1. Start by heating your oven to 375.
2. Rub a nine inch pie dish down with your rosemary olive oil.
3. Bleat your eggs in a bowl before stirring in your cream cheese, heavy cream, rosemary, salt and ham, making sure it's mixed well.
4. Pour the mixture into your pie dish, and then bake until your eggs are set to a golden brown. This will take about a half hour.
5. Let your quiche rest before serving.

Raspberry & Chocolate Cheesecake Shake

Serves: 1

Calories: 251

Fat: 15 Grams

Protein: 25 Grams

Fiber: 5 Grams

Net Carbs: 4 Grams

Time: 5 Minutes

Ingredients:

- 1 Cup Almond Milk, Unsweetened
- 1 Tablespoon Heavy Whipping Cream
- 1 Tablespoon Cream Cheese
- ½ Cup Raspberries, Fresh
- 2 Ice Cubes
- 1/3 Cup Vanilla Whey Protein Powder

Directions:

1. Blend together until smooth before serving.

Peanut Butter & Chocolate Smoothie

Serves: 1

Calories: 604

Fat: 49 Grams

Protein: 33 Grams

Fiber: 2 rams

Net Carbs: 6 Grams

Time: 5 Minutes

Ingredients:

- 1/3 Cup Low Carb Chocolate Whey Protein Powder
- 2 Ice Cubes
- 2 tablespoons Peanut Butter, Unsweetened
- 1 Cup Water
- ½ Cup Heavy Whipping Cream

Directions:

1. Blend well before serving.

Sage & Strawberry Smoothie

Serves: 1

Calories: 173

Fat: 16 Gras

Protein: 2 Grams

Fiber: 1 Gram

Net Carbs: 5 Grams

Time: 5 Minutes

Ingredients:

- 5 Strawberries, Frozen
- 2 Tablespoons Heavy Whipping Cream
- 1 Cup Coconut Milk, Unsweetened
- 1 Fresh Sage Leaf
- 1 Teaspoon Vanilla Bean Sweetener

Directions:

1. Blend until smooth before serving.

Chapter 6: Lunch Recipes

When you're going keto, there are many soups and salads to choose from as well as other lunch recipes. Still, keep in mind that this is a great time to get the fiber you need, especially if you're trying to alleviate the keto flu.

Keto Caesar Salad

Serves: 4

Calories: 727

Fat: 38.75

Net Carbs: 1.8 Grams

Fiber: 0.5 Grams

Protein: 13 Grams

Time: 15 Minutes

Ingredients:

- 4 Tablespoons Shaved Parmesan
- 2 Ounces Pork Rinds, Chopped Small
- 24 Whole Leaves Romaine Hearts
- 2 Garlic Cloves, Minced
- 4 Tablespoons Grated Parmesan
- 4 Anchovy Fillets
- 1 Teaspoon Dijon Mustard
- 8 Tablespoons Avocado Oil
- 1 Egg Yolk
- 3 Tablespoons Apple Cider Vinegar

Directions:

1. Blend your apple cider vinegar, egg yolk, and mustard in a blender. Pour the avocado oil on top. Blend on low.
2. Add in your garlic, grated parmesan and anchovies.
3. Blend on slow until it creates a smooth dressing.
4. Drizzle on your leaves, and then divide your pork rinds between servings. Garnish with your shaved parmesan.

Pizza Bread

Serves: 12

Calories: 175

Fiber: 4 Grams

Protein: 12 Grams

Fat: 12.5 Grams

Net Carbs: 1.9 Grams

Time: 45 Minutes

Ingredients:

- ¼ Teaspoon Sea Salt, Fine
- 1/3 Cup Flax meal
- 1 Teaspoon Cream of Tartar
- ½ Teaspoon Baking Soda
- ¼ Cup Psyllium Husk Powder
- 1 Cup Parmesan Cheese, Grated Fine
- 1 Teaspoon Ghee
- 4 Egg Whites, Large
- ½ Cup Water, Lukewarm
- ½ Cup Marinara Sauce
- 1 Cup Mozzarella Cheese, Shredded
- 4.2 Ounces Pepperoni, Diced

Directions:

1. Heat your oven to 350, and mix your ½ cup of marinara with your egg whites and water.
2. Dice your pepperoni, and set it to the side.
3. Combine all of your dry ingredients together, and then put a medium skillet over heat. It's best to use a cast iron oven safe skillet.
4. Pour your marinara into the mixture, and process in a food processor before adding in your pepperoni.
5. Make twelve buns, placing each in your skillet.
6. Transfer your pan into the oven, baking for twenty-five to thirty minutes.
7. Top with your mozzarella cheese, and bake for another five minutes. The cheese should melt and become crisp.
8. Take it out of the oven, letting it cool down before serving.

Spinach Tabbouleh

Serves: 6

Calories: 245

Fiber: 3 Grams

Protein: 2.6 Grams

Fat: 23.5 Grams

Net Carbs: 5.4 Grams

Time: 20 Minutes

Ingredients:

- 2 Tablespoons Extra Virgin Coconut Oil
- 3 Cups Cauliflower Rice
- 1 Clove Garlic, Minced
- ½ Cup Extra Virgin Olive Oil
- ½ Cup Lemon Juice, Fresh
- ½ Cup Mint, Fresh & Chopped
- ¼ Teaspoon Black Pepper
- 3 Cups Spinach, Chopped
- 1 Cup Parsley, Fresh & Chopped
- 2 Spring Onions, Medium & Chopped
- 1 Medium Cucumber, Diced & Peeled
- 1 Cup Cherry Tomatoes, Chopped
- 1 Teaspoon Sea Salt, Fine

Directions:

1. Heat a pan with your coconut oil using medium heat.
2. Add your cauliflower rice, seasoning with salt. Coo it for five minutes, and then let it cool.
3. Place your chopped vegetables in a salad bowl, adding in your mint and parsley.
4. Chop your spinach and add it into your cooling cauliflower rice.
5. Juice your lemons, pouring it into a bowl before mixing in your olive oil and garlic, whisking.
6. Pour it over your vegetables, and mix everything together before serving.

Butternut & Turkey Soup

Serves: 8

Calories: 108

Fiber: 0 Grams

Protein: 6 Grams

Fat: 7.5 Grams

Net Carbs: 3.25 Grams

Total Time: 9 Hours 15 Minutes

Ingredients:

- 1 Carrot, Medium
- 1 Tablespoon Sea Salt, Fine
- 1 Teaspoon Peppercorns, Whole
- 2-3 Legs Celery
- 1 Tablespoon Apple Cider Vinegar, Organic
- 2-3 Turkey Necks
- 1 Turkey Carcass
- ½ Teaspoon Ginger Powder
- ½ Teaspoon Turmeric Powder
- 1 Cup Butternut Squash, Cubed & Peeled
- 4 Ounces Turkey Meat (From Turkey Necks)

Directions:

1. Start by submerging your turkey parts and vegetables with a gallon of water, and then add in your apple cider vinegar and sea salt.
2. Bring it to a boil, simmering for eight hours.
3. After four hours, remove the necks and all of the meat. Return the bones to the pot.
4. Set the meat aside, as it can keep in the refrigerator for a week.
5. Drain the stock to get the bone out, and then place your stock in a clean pot. Add in your turmeric and garlic.
6. Let it simmer for an hour, and then filter again.
7. Add two quarts of your stock to your cubed butternut squash. Let it simmer for a half hour until your squash turns tender. Add in your turkey meat, and simmer for another ten minutes.

8. Serve warm.

Greek Salad

Serves: 4

Calories: 323

Fiber: 3.3 Grams

Protein: 9.3 Grams

Fat: 27.8 Grams

Net Carbs: 8 Grams

Time: 10 Minutes

Ingredients:

- 4 Tablespoons Extra Virgin Olive Oil
- Salt & Pepper to Taste
- 7.1 Ounces Feta Cheese
- 1 Teaspoon Oregano, Dried
- 16 Olives
- 4 Tablespoons Capers
- 1 Red Onion, Small
- 1 Green Pepper, Medium
- 1 Cucumber, Large
- 4-5 Tomatoes

Directions:

1. Wash your tomatoes before slicing.
2. Peel your cucumber and then slice.
3. Deseed and half your green pepper, slicing.
4. Peel your onion before slicing, and then place everything in a bowl.
5. Add your oregano, olives and capers.
6. Add in your feta, and drizzle with your olive oil before serving.

Brussels Salad

Serves: 1

Calories: 282

Fat: 28 Grams

Protein: 3 Gras

Fiber: 3 Grams

Net Carbs: 5 Grams

Time: 5 Minutes

Ingredients:

- 1 Cup Brussels Sprouts, Chopped
- 2 Tablespoons Olive Oil
- 1 Tablespoon Lemon Juice, Fresh
- ¼ Teaspoon Black Pepper

Directions:

1. Toss together before serving. Many people prefer to slice their Brussel sprouts in half first, but it's up to preference.

Pesto Gnocchi

Serves: 4

Calories: 720

Fat: 60 Grams

Protein: 42 Grams

Fiber: 2 Grams

Net Carbs: 7 Grams

Time: 40 Minutes

Ingredients:

- 1 Cup Basil Leaves, Fresh
- 2 Tablespoons Pine Nuts
- 2 Garlic Cloves, Peeled
- ¼ Teaspoon Nutmeg, Ground
- ¼ Cup + 2 Teaspoons Olive Oil, Divided
- 1 Brazil Nut
- 1/3 Cup Parmesan Cheese, Grated
- 4 Cups Mozzarella Cheese, Shredded
- 3 Tablespoons Golden Ghee
- 5 Egg Yolks, Large
- 5 Grape Tomatoes

Directions:

1. Grind your basil, pine nuts, Brazil nuts, garlic, olive oil and nutmeg together to make a pesto. Mix in your parmesan, and then set it aside.
2. Microwave your mozzarella until melted in thirty second intervals, and then add in your egg yolks, kneading until it turns dough like.
3. Roll the dough out in one foot long rolls, refrigerating for ten minutes.
4. Bring a pot of water to a boil, and make sure to salt it.
5. Cut your rolls into inch pieces using a knife, and then drop in the boiling water. Cook for three minutes before draining.
6. Melt your ghee over medium-high heat, and then add in your gnocchi. Fry until crispy on both sides, which takes about a minute.
7. In another skillet, add in two teaspoons olive oil, cooking over medium heat, and then add in your tomatoes. Stir in your pesto once softened, cooking for about another minute.
8. Pour this sauce over your gnocchi, tossing until combined.

Blue Cheese Zoodles

Serves: 1

Calories: 435

Fat: 33 Grams

Protein: 21 Grams

Fiber: 1 Gram

Net Carbs: 5 Grams

Time: 10 Minutes

Ingredients:

- ½ Cup Baby Spinach
- 1/3 Cup Blue Cheese, Crumbled
- 3 Tablespoons Blue Cheese Dressing, Chunky
- ¼ Teaspoon Black Pepper
- ½ Cup Bacon, Cooked & Crumbled
- 1 Cup Zucchini, Spiralized

Directions:

1. Toss together until combined, serving cold.

Tricolore Salad

Serves: 2

Calories: 581

Fiber: 9 Grams

Protein: 19.2 Grams

Fat: 50.7 Grams

Net Carbs: 8.6 Grams

Time: 10 Minutes

Ingredients:

- 2 Tablespoons Extra Virgin Olive Oil
- 2 Tablespoons Pesto
- Salt & Pepper to Taste
- 4.4 Ounces Mozzarella
- 6-8 Olives
- 1 Avocado, Large
- 3-4 Tomatoes

Directions:

1. Start by washing your tomatoes off before slicing.
2. Deseed, halve and peel your avocado before slicing.
3. Deseed your olives and cut them in half, and place your tomatoes, avocado and olives in a bowl.
4. Crumble your mozzarella, adding it to the bowl.
5. Add in your pesto and olive oil, and season with salt and pepper before serving.

Seasoned Turnip Fries

Serves: 4

Calories: 129

Fiber: 3.3 Grams

Protein: 1.7 Grams

Fat: 9.5 Grams

Net Carbs: 7.7 Grams

Time: 35 Minutes

Ingredients:

- 2 lbs Turnips
- 2 Teaspoons Sea Salt, Fine
- 2 Tablespoons Taco Seasoning
- ¼ Cup Light Olive Oil

Directions:

1. Start by heating your oven to 350.
2. Wash your turnips before patting them dry. Peel them before slicing into fries.
3. Place them in a bowl, drizzling your olive oil, salt and taco seasoning over them, tossing to combine.
4. Line a baking sheet with parchment paper, and then place your turnips on it in a single layer.
5. Bake for about twenty-five minutes or until golden brown. Let cool before serving.

Salmon Poke Bowl

Serves: 2

Calories: 558

Fiber: 8.8 Grams

Protein: 30.3 Grams

Fat: 42.4 Grams

Net Carbs: 8.5 Grams

Time: 25 Minutes

Ingredients:

- ½ lb Sushi Grade Salmon, Boneless & Skinless
- 2 Tablespoons Coconut Aminos
- 1 Teaspoon Sriracha Sauce
- 2 Medium Green Onions, Chopped
- 1 Tablespoon Sesame Seeds
- ½ Teaspoon Sea Salt, Fine
- 1 Teaspoon Rice Vinegar
- 1 Tablespoon Lemon Juice, Fresh
- 1 Tablespoon Sesame Oil, Toasted

Cauliflower Rice:

- ¼ Teaspoon Sea Salt
- 1 Tablespoon Rice Vinegar
- Tablespoon Ghee
- 2 Cups Cauliflower Rice

Toppings:

- 1 Avocado, Seeded & Peeled
- 1 Tablespoon Ghee
- Salt to Taste
- 1 Nori Seaweed Sheet

Directions:

1. Start by marinating your salmon. You'll need to mix your vinegar, lemon juice, toasted sesame oil, coconut aminos and salt together. Cut into one inch pieces, mixing in a bowl.
2. Add your marinade to your sesame seeds and green onions.

3. Add your sriracha, and then mix well.
4. Grate your cauliflower rice in a food processor, and then grease a pan with your ghee. Cook for five to seven minutes over medium-high heat.
5. Take off of heat, and then mix in your vinegar.
6. Crisp your nori pieces in a hot pan with ghee.
7. Slice your avocado, and then place your rice in the bowl. Add in your salmon. Add in your nori and avocado.

Ricotta & Lemon Zoodles

Serves: 2

Calories: 181

Fiber: 4 Grams

Fat: 12 Grams

Protein: 9 Grams

Net Carbs: 4 Grams

Time: 15 Minutes

Ingredients:

- ½ Cup Ricotta Cheese
- 1 Small Lemon, Grated for Zest
- ½ Shallot, Minced
- ½ Teaspoon Sea Salt, Fine
- ¼ Teaspoon Black Pepper
- 4 Chard Leaves, Chopped & Stemmed
- 1 Tablespoon Golden Ghee
- 2 Cups Zucchini, Spiralized
- 1 ½ Teaspoons Thyme Leaves, Fresh

Directions:

1. Mix your ricotta cheese, salt, pepper, and zest together before setting aside.
2. Take a skillet and melt your ghee over medium heat, and then add in your chard. Sauté until the chard is softened, which should take one to two minutes. Add in your shallots, cooking for another minute.
3. Stir in your zucchini noodles and thyme. Cook for about one more minute, and then stir in your ricotta mix, cooking for another two minutes.

Egg Drop Soup

Serves: 6

Calories: 255

Fiber: 0.8 Grams

Protein: 10.8 Grams

Fat: 22.4 Grams

Net Carbs: 2.9 Grams

Time: 20 Minutes

Ingredients:

- 2 Quarts Chicken Stock
- 1 Tablespoon Turmeric, Grated
- 1 Tablespoon Ginger, Grated
- 6 Tablespoons Extra Virgin Olive Oil
- Salt & Pepper to Taste
- 2 Spring Onions, Sliced
- 2 Tablespoons Cilantro, Freshly Chopped
- 4 Eggs, Large
- 4 Cups Swiss Chard, Chopped
- 2 Tablespoons Coconut aminos
- 2 Cups Brown Mushrooms, Sliced
- 1 Small Chile Pepper, Sliced
- 2 Garlic Cloves, Chopped

Directions:

1. Grate your ginger root, grate your turmeric and then slice your chile peppers. Mince your garlic cloves.
2. Pour your chicken stock in a pot, and heat over medium heat. Let it simmer while you slice your mushrooms.
3. Slice your chard, and then place your chile pepper, ginger, turmeric, garlic, chard stalks, mushrooms, and coconut aminos in a pot, simmering for five minutes.
4. Add your chard leaves, cooking for another minute.
5. Whisk in your eggs, pouring them into the soup while it's at a simmer.
6. Stir until your egg is cooked, and then take the pot off of heat.

7. Cop your cilantro and spring onions, adding them and then seasoning with salt and pepper.
8. Pour into serving bowls before drizzling with extra virgin olive oil if you desire.

Duck Ramen

Serves: 4

Calories: 542

Fiber: 3.9 Grams

Protein: 34.4 Grams

Fat: 40.2 Grams

Net Carbs: 7.1 Grams

Time: 40 Minutes

Ingredients:

- 2 Duck Breasts, Sin on
- 4 Spring Onions, Sliced (Separate the White & Green Parts)
- 1 Bunch Swiss Chard
- 2 Tablespoons Ginger, Grated
- 2 Cups Shiitake Mushrooms, Sliced
- 1 Small Chili Pepper, Slice & Deseeded
- 2 Tablespoons Fish Sauce
- 2 Tablespoons Coconut Aminos
- 6 Cups Chicken Stock
- 4 Duck Eggs, Medium
- 1 lb Kelp Noodles, Drained
- Salt & Pepper to Taste
- 2 Teaspoons Sesame Seeds
- 2 Teaspoons Sesame Seed Oil
- 2 Teaspoons Extra Virgin Olive Oil
- 4 Teaspoons Sriracha Sauce

Directions:

1. Turn your oven to 425.
2. Pat your duck skin down with a paper towel in order to remove moisture. Score the side with the skin, seasoning with salt and pepper.

3. Heat a pan over medium-high heat, placing the skin side down onto the hot pan. You won't need oil.
4. Pour the fat over the breasts as it's released, cooking for six to eight minutes. It should turn lightly golden, and then turn it. Cook for another thirty seconds.
5. Take a roasting tin with a rack, and place the skin side up, transferring your duck onto it and into the oven. Cook for fifteen minutes if you want medium-rare, and reserve some duck fat for cooing later.
6. Rest the meat in a warm place for ten minutes. Do not cover it, and then slice.
7. Pour your duck fat into a large pot, adding in your white parts of the onion, ginger, and chili pepper. Cook until fragrant.
8. Chop your chard, and then place the stalks into the pot, cooing for three to five minutes. Keep your chard leaves separate for now.
9. Add your fish sauce, chopped chard leaves, coconut aminos and chicken stocks into the pot, bringing it all to a boil. You'll need to use high eat, and then once it starts to simmer reduce it to medium.
10. Add in your mushrooms, cooking for five minutes.
11. Add in your kelp noodles, turning the heat off. Season with salt and pepper to taste.
12. Place your eggs in a pot of water, and then bring to a boil over high heat. Cook for seven to eight minutes. Peel them, and then half them.
13. Pour your soup into bowls, which should take about two cups for each serving.
14. Top with sliced duck breasts, green parts of your onions, and one egg half per serving, sesame seeds, sesame oil, olive oil and sriracha. Serve hot.

Cheesy Baked Zoodles

Serves: 6

Calories: 655

Fat: 54 Grams

Protein: 35 Grams

Fiber: 2 Grams

Net Carbs: 6 Grams

Time: 1 Hour 15 Minutes

Ingredients:

- 1 ½ Tablespoons Sea Salt, Fine
- Golden Ghee
- 2 Cps Monetary Jack Cheese, Grated
- 4 Cups Cheddar Cheese, Grated
- ¼ Cup Heavy Whipping Cream
- ¼ Teaspoon Garlic Powder
- 4 Tablespoons Salted Butter, Room Temperature
- 4 Eggs, Large
- ¾ Cup Almond Milk, Unsweetened
- 6 Zucchini, Large & Spiralized

Directions:

1. Start by heating your oven to 350, and then grease a ten inch pie dish using your golden ghee.
2. Sat your zucchini and let it sit for fifteen minutes before patting dry with a paper towel. Lay it on fresh paper towels to continue drying. This will remove excess liquid.
3. Whisk your almond milk, eggs, heavy cream, garlic powder and butter together in a bowl.
4. Layer your zucchini noodles into your pie dish, and then cover with your cheeses. Mix together, and then pour your egg mixture over your zoodles.
5. Bake for thirty-five to forty-five minutes. Cut into wedges before serving.

Vietnamese Pho

Serves: 4

Calories: 294

Fiber: 2.1 Grams

Protein: 32.3 Grams

Fat: 15.6 Grams

Net Carbs: 6.5 Grams

Time: 30 Minutes

Ingredients:

- 4" Piece Ginger Root, Peeled
- 1 White Onion, Medium & Quartered
- 8 Cups Beef Broth
- 1 lb Beef, Sliced Thin
- 14.1 Ounces Shirataki Noodles
- 1 Tablespoon Coconut Aminos
- 1 Tablespoon Fish Sauce
- 2 Cloves Garlic, Crushed
- Green Onions, Sliced for Topping
- Bean Sprouts for Topping

Directions:

1. Place your beef in the freezer for twenty minutes to slice.
2. Char the onions and ginger for five to seven minutes in a broiler.
3. Add them to a large soup pot, adding in your fish sauce, garlic and coconut aminos.
4. Pour your broth in, and then turn the heat to medium-high, bringing it to a boil.
5. Reduce to simmer, cooking for a half hour. Raise the heat, bringing to a boil.
6. While your broth is cooing, prepare your noodles according to package instructions.
7. Place your beef in bowls, and then pour the noodles and broth on top. You should notice your beef starts to brown.
8. Top with desired toppings.

Chapter 7: Snack Recipes

If you're on a keto diet, you'll need to have snacks two times a day. You'll need it once after breakfast and once after lunch. Here are some salt and savory snacks for you to try.

Goat Cheese & Roasted Tomato

Serves: 2

Calories: 101

Fat: 8 Grams

Protein: 6 Grams

Fiber: 2 Grams

Net Carbs: 2 Grams

Time: 35 Minutes

Ingredients:

- 2 Plum Tomatoes
- ½ Teaspoon Sea Salt, Fine
- 2 Tablespoons Caramelized Onions
- Extra Virgin Olive Oil
- 4 Tablespoons Goat Cheese, Crumbled & Divided
- 1 Teaspoon Thyme Leaves, Fresh & Divided

Directions:

1. Start by heating your oven to 425.
2. Halve your tomatoes lengthwise, removing pulp as well as the seeds.
3. Place them with the cut side down on your baking sheet, and then drizzle with olive oil.
4. Add ½ tablespoon of caramelized onions to your tomatoes at the bottom, and then add a tablespoon of goat cheese to each one. Sprinkle thyme on top.
5. Bake for thirty minutes before serving.

Bacon Fat Bombs

Serves: 12

Calories: 89

Fat: 8 Grams

Protein: 3 Grams

Fiber: 0 Grams

Net Carbs: 0 Grams

Time: 1 Hour 10 Minutes

Ingredients:

- 2 Ounces Cream Cheese, Room Temperature
- 2 Ounces Goat Cheese, Room Temperature
- ¼ Cup Butter, Room Temperature
- 8 Bacon Slices, Chopped & Cooked
- Black Pepper to Taste

Directions:

1. Line a baking sheet with parchment paper.
2. Take your cream cheese, goat cheese, bacon and pepper, combining it together.
3. Use a tablespoon and drop these bombs on the baking sheet. Freeze until firm. This should take an hour, but make sure they aren't completely frozen.
4. Store in a sealed container in the fridge for up to two weeks.

Creamy Deviled Eggs

Serves: 6

Calories: 202

Fat: 15 Grams

Protein: 14 Gras

Fiber: 0 Grams

Net Carbs: 3 Grams

Time: 40 Minutes

Ingredients:

- 12 Eggs, Large
- 6 Tablespoons Mayonnaise
- 1 Teaspoon Sea Salt, Fine
- 1 Tablespoon Dill, Dried

Directions:

1. Place each egg while it's whole in mini muffin tins, and then turn your oven to 325. Place in the oven, baking for thirty minutes.
2. Transfer your eggs to a bowl of ice water, and then peel each egg before cutting in half lengthwise. Scoop the yolk out, reserving the yolk in a small bowl.
3. Add in your dill, mayonnaise and salt into your yolks, mixing until smooth.
4. Place the yolk mixture into your eggs, and serve cool.

Salmon Fat Bombs

Serves: 12

Calories: 193

Protein: 8 Grams

Fiber: 0 Grams

Net Carbs: 0 Grams

Time: 2 Hours 10 Minutes

Ingredients:

- ½ Cup Goat Cheese, Room Temperature
- Black Pepper to taste
- 2 Teaspoon Lemon Juice, Fresh
- 2 Ounces Smoked Salmon
- ½ Cup Butter, Room Temperature

Directions:

1. Line a baking sheet with parchment paper.
2. Tae a bowl and stir together your butter, salon, goat cheese, pepper and lemon juice. Make sure it's blended well.
3. Use a tablespoon to place twelve even mounds on the baking sheet, and put it in the fridge for two to three hours.
4. Store in an airtight container, and it'll keep in the fridge for one full week.

Crab Dip

Serves: 4-6

Calories: 292

Fat: 31 Grams

Protein: 21 Grams

Fiber: 0 Grams

Net Carbs: 2 Grams

Time: 40 Minutes

Ingredients:

- 1 lb Crabmeat, Lump
- Butter, Room Temperature
- ½ Cup Red Bell Pepper, Diced
- 2 Teaspoons Cajun Seasoning
- 1 Tablespoon Horseradish
- 1 Tablespoon Mayonnaise
- 1 Cup Cream Cheese, Room Temperature
- 1/8 Teaspoon Garlic Salt

Directions:

1. Heat your oven to 350, and then grease a baking dish with butter.
2. Mix your red bell pepper, cream cheese, crabmeat, horseradish, Cajun seasoning, garlic and mayonnaise together until blended well.
3. Transfer to a baking dish, baking for thirty minutes. Serve warm with celery ribs.

Parmesan Chips

Serves: 4

Calories: 228

Fat: 15 Grams

Protein: 23 Grams

Fiber: 0 Grams

Net Carbs: 2 Grams

Time: 10 Minutes

Ingredients:

- ½ Teaspoon Sea Salt, Fine
- 10 Ounces Parmesan Cheese, Shredded

Directions:

1. Start by heating your oven to 350.
2. Line a baking sheet using parchment paper, and then form parmesan cheese circles on each sheet.
3. Bake until brown. This takes three to five minutes.
4. Sprinkle with salt before letting it cool to serve.

Walnut & Herb Goat Cheese

Serves: 4

Calories: 304

Fat: 28 Grams

Protein: 12 Grams

Fiber: 2 Grams

Net Carbs: 2 Grams

Time: 10 Minutes

Ingredients:

- 1 Tablespoon Oregano, Chopped
- 1 Teaspoon Thyme, Fresh & Chopped
- 6 Ounces Walnuts, Chopped
- 1 Teaspoon Thyme, Fresh & Chopped
- ¼ Teaspoon Black Pepper
- 8 Ounces Goat Cheese

Directions:

1. Place your parsley, thyme, oregano, walnuts and pepper in a food processor. Pulse until chopped fine.
2. Pour the mixture into the goat cheese, and then roll it in the nut mixture.
3. Wrap and refrigerate for one week.

Sour Cream Pork Rinds

Serves: 4-6

Calories: 278

Fiber: 0 Grams

Fat: 19 Grams

Protein: 25 Grams

Net Carbs: 1.5 Grams

Time: 2 Hours 50 Minutes

Ingredients:

- 2 lbs Pork Skin
- 2 Tablespoons Onion Powder
- 1 Tablespoon Garlic Powder
- 3 Tablespoons Sweet Cream Buttermilk Powder
- 3 Tablespoons Chives

Directions:

1. Start by heating your oven to 350.
2. Cut your pork skin into one inch pieces, and then put them skin side up on your baking sheets.
3. Bake your skins for two and a half hours, and then remove from the baking sheet. Let it cool before handling.
4. Toss them in a bowl with your buttermilk powder, chives, onion powder and garlic powder.
5. You can serve at room temperature or warm.

Roasted Almonds

Serves: 8

Calories: 229

Fiber: 5.1 Grams

Protein: 8 Grams

Fat: 19.6 Gras

Net Carbs: 4.3 Grams

Time: 13 Hours

Ingredients:

- 2 Cups Almonds, Raw
- 1 Tablespoon Paprika
- 1 Tablespoon Olive Oil
- 1 Teaspoon Pepper
- 1 Teaspoon Garlic Powder
- 1 Teaspoon Cumin
- 2 Teaspoon Sea Salt, Fine
- 2 Teaspoons Chili Powder
- 1 Teaspoon Onion Powder

Directions:

1. Start by placing your almonds in a jar, covering with water. They'll need to soak for twelve hours.
2. Drain your excess water, patting them dry with paper towels.
3. Heat your oven to 300, and then take a baking sheet, lining it with parchment paper.
4. Toss your almonds in a bowl with your spices and olive oil, spreading the almonds on the baking sheet in a single layer.
5. Place in the oven, cooking for forty-five minutes. Make sure to stir occasionally. When they're done they should be crunchy and dry.

Beef Jerky

Yields: 8 Slices

Serving Size: 2 Slices

Calories: 161

Fiber: 0.1 Grams

Protein: 10.8 Grams

Fat: 12.5 Grams

Net Carbs: 0.4 Grams

Time: 5-6 Hours

Ingredients:

- 1.1 lb Lean Beef, Minced
- 1 Teaspoon Sea Salt
- 1 Tablespoon Coconut Aminos
- ½ Teaspoon Onion Powder
- ½ Teaspoon Paprika
- ½ Teaspoon Black Pepper
- ½ Teaspoon Garlic Powder

Directions:

1. Mix all ingredients together in a bowl.
2. Place the meat on parchment paper, and then roll out the meat. It should be ¼ inch thick.
3. Cut into sixteen pieces.
4. Heat your oven to 190, and then cook for four to five hours. The meat should be dry. You'll need to drain the juices every two hours. Flip your jerky halfway through.
5. Let cool before serving.

Chapter 8: Dinner Dishes

You'll need dinner when you're on the keto diet even if they aren't heavy. With your snacks, a light dinner is usually good enough to keep you full.

Skillet Salmon

Serves: 2-4

Calories: 684

Fat: 47 Grams

Protein: 67 Grams

Fiber: 1 Gram

Net Carbs: 1 Grams

Time: 20 Minutes

Ingredients:

- 1 Tablespoon Garlic, Minced
- 4 Tablespoons Golden Ghee, Divided
- ½ Teaspoon Sea Salt, Fine
- 1 Shallot, Quartered
- ¼ Lemon
- 4 Salmon Fillets, 6 Ounces

Directions:

1. Start by heating your oven to 450, and then mix two tablespoons of ghee with thyme, garlic and salt together. Set this bowl aside.
2. Take a medium cast iron skillet, and then melt your remaining two tablespoons of ghee.
3. Add in your salmon fillets, making sure the skin side is down.
4. Wedge your shallots between each salmon fillet, and then sear for one minute on one side. Flip, and then sear for another minute.
5. Brea your shallot quarters, and then top your salmon with your seasoning.
6. Transfer your skillet into your oven before baking for eight minutes.
7. Serve with roasted shallots and fresh lemon juice.

Coconut & Lime Steak

Serves: 2-3

Calories: 1,182

Fiber: 1 Grams

Protein: 121 Grams

Fat: 73 Grams

Net Carbs: 3 Grams

Time: 40 minutes

Ingredients:

- ¼ Cup Coconut Oil, Melted
- 2 Tablespoons Lime Juice, Fresh
- Zest of 1 Lime
- 1 Tablespoon Garlic, Minced
- 1 Teaspoon Sea Salt, Fine
- 2 lbs Skirt Steak
- 1 Teaspoon Red Pepper Flakes
- 1 Teaspoon Ginger, Grated Fresh

Directions:

1. Combine your lime juice, lime zest, coconut toil, ginger, garlic, salt and red pepper flakes together. Add in your steak, coating it before letting it marinate for twenty minutes. Do not put it in the fridge.
2. Transfer to a skillet, and cook over medium-high heat. If you have to cut it, make sure to cut it against the grain.
3. Sear on both sides, and then cook as desired. Slice before serving warm.

Keto Baked Haddock

Serves: 4

Calories: 477

Fiber: 2 Grams

Protein: 56 Grams

Fat: 23 Grams

Net Carbs: 7 Grams

Time: 55 Minutes

Ingredients:

- 1 lb Bulk Sausage
- 2 Tablespoons Sage, Fresh & Chopped
- 1 Tablespoon Lemon Zest, Grated
- ½ Teaspoon Sea Salt, Fine
- ¼ Teaspoon Black Pepper
- 2 Tablespoon Lemon Juice, Fresh & Divided
- 4 Haddock Fillets, 6-7 Ounces Each
- 1 Tablespoon Garlic, Minced
- 2 Tablespoon Garlic Infused Olive Oil
- 1 Onion, Medium & Quartered
- 10 Cherry Tomatoes, Halved
- 1 Cup Fennel, Sliced Thin

Directions:

1. Start by heating your oven to 400.
2. Take an oven proof skillet, cooking your sage and sausage over medium-high heat. You'll want to brown your meat and make sure it's thoroughly cooked, stirring often. Break it into large clumps, which will take about five minutes.
3. Remove from the skillet, but leave your rendered fat in the skillet. Set the sausage asides.
4. Add your fennel to the skillet, and top with onion and tomatoes. Drizzle your garlic olive oil on it, and season with salt and pepper. Add in a tablespoon of lemon juice over your vegetables, and then place in the oven for thirty minutes. You'll need to stir occasionally.

5. Mix the remaining tablespoon of lemon juice, lemon zest and minced garlic together, tossing your haddock fillets in the mix before setting your fillet aside.
6. Once your vegetables are roasted, add in your sausage, and then place your haddock fillets on top.
7. Bake for another ten minutes before serving warm.

Cheesy Italian Meatballs

Serves: 5

Calories: 521

Fiber: 0 Grams

Protein: 72 Grams

Fat: 23 Grams

Net Carbs: 4 Grams

Time: 40 Minutes

Ingredients:

- 1 lb Ground Pork
- 1 lb Ground Beef
- 1 Tablespoon Water
- 1 Egg, Large & Lightly Beaten
- ½ Cup Parmesan Cheese, Grated
- ½ Cup Mozzarella Cheese, Shredded
- 1 Teaspoon Cajun Seasoning
- 1 Tablespoon Italian Seasoning
- 1 Teaspoon Sea Salt, Fine
- 1 Tablespoon Garlic, Minced
- 1 Teaspoon Black Pepper
- 8 Ounces Mozzarella Cheese

Directions:

1. Start by heating your oven to 400.
2. Line a baking sheet with parchment paper.
3. Combine your pork, egg, water, beef, mozzarella, parmesan, Italian seasoning, garlic, Cajun seasoning, salt and pepper together in a bowl, mixing well.
4. Form into meat balls, and then cut your mozzarella into cubes. Make sure you have one cube for each meatball you made.
5. Stuff a cube into the middle of your meatballs and then re-seal them.
6. Place your meatballs on the baking sheet, baking for twenty minutes. They should be cooked all the way through, and then serve hot.

Coffee Tuna Steak

Serves: 2

Calories: 241

Fat: 10 Grams

Protein: 34 Grams

Fiber: 1 Gram

Net Carbs: 2 Grams

Time: 40 Minutes

Ingredients:

- Extra Virgin Olive Oil
- 2 Tuna Steaks, 4 Ounces Each
- 1 Tablespoon Black Pepper
- 3 Tablespoon Ground Coffee, Fine
- 1 Teaspoon Sea Salt, Fine
- ½ Teaspoon Ground Cinnamon
- ½ Teaspoon Chili Powder

Directions:

1. Start by brushing your tuna down with olive oil.
2. Take a bowl, combining your pepper, salt, coffee, cinnamon and chili powder together.
3. Sprinkle this mix over your tuna steaks on both sides, letting them rest for a half hour.
4. Brush your tuna down with more olive oil and sear them in a pan over high heat. Cook until done and serve hot.

Vegetable Fried Beef

Serves: 4

Calories: 297

Fat: 13 Grams

Protein: 42 Grams

Fiber: 2 Grams

Net Carbs: 3 Grams

Time: 20 Minutes

Ingredients:

- 1 lb Ground Beef
- 1 Tablespoon Tamari
- 1 Tablespoon Peanut Butter
- 3 Eggs, Medium
- 1 Cup Pea Pods, Trimmed
- 1/8 Teaspoon Ground Ginger
- 1 Scallion, Chopped
- ¼ Cup Broccoli, Chopped

Directions:

1. Brown your beef in a medium skillet over medium-high heat, cooking for about three minutes. Remove from your pan, and then leave some grease in the skillet. You don't need all of your grease.
2. Crack your eggs into the skillet, and then stir until cooked and scrambled.
3. Return your meat to the skillet, and then stir in your pea pods, broccoli, ginger, peanut butter and scallion.
4. Cover and cook for five more minutes, stirring and then serve warm.

Wrapped Tilapia

Serves: 2-4

Calories: 788

Fiber: 0 Grams

Protein: 94 Grams

Fat: 47 Grams

Net Carbs: 2 Grams

Time: 40 Minutes

Ingredients:

- 4 Tilapia Fillets, Rinsed & Patted Dry (6 Ounces Each)
- 3 Tablespoons Golden Ghee
- Black Pepper to taste
- 1 Teaspoon Basil, Dried
- 1 ½ Tablespoon Lemon Juice, Fresh
- ¼ Cup Mayonnaise
- 12 Bacon Strips

Directions:

1. Start by heating your oven to 375.
2. Line a baking sheet with parchment paper, and then brush your tilapia down with your ghee. Sprinkle with basil and pepper, and then wrap your fillets with bacon.
3. Bake for twenty to thirty minutes.
4. While its baking whisk your lemon juice, more pepper, and mayonnaise together. Serve this on top of your fish once done.

Beef Roll Ups

Serves: 4

Calories: 527

Fat: 27 Grams

Protein: 66 Grams

Fiber: 1 Gram

Net Carbs: 1 Gram

Time: 1 Hour 10 Minutes

Ingredients:

- 1 Tablespoons Olive Oil
- 2 Teaspoon Garlic, Minced
- 1 Teaspoon Sea Salt, Fine
- 1/8 Teaspoon Ground Cinnamon
- 1 Teaspoon Black Pepper
- 2 Teaspoon Rosemary Leaves, Chopped Fresh
- 2 Teaspoon Thyme Leaves, Chopped Fresh
- 2 lbs Flank Steak, Pounded Thin & Cut into Pieces (4x4 Inches)
- ½ Cup Blue Cheese, Crumbled

Directions:

1. Start by heating your oven to 375, and then line a baking sheet with parchment paper.
2. Soak ten to twenty toothpicks in water.
3. Take a bowl and combine your garlic, olive oil, rosemary, thyme, cinnamon, salt and pepper together, putting it in a plastic bag.
4. Add in your steak, marinating for thirty minutes.
5. Lay on a sheet, and then put blue cheese in the middle of each.
6. Roll them up, and then put your damp toothpicks through the roll.
7. Bake for ten to twenty minutes until they reach your desired doneness, and then serve warm.

Goat Cheese Burgers

Serves: 2

Calories: 857

Protein: 48.9 Grams

Fat: 33.6 Grams

Fiber: 1.4 Grams

Net Carbs: 7.3 Grams

Time: 20 Minutes

Ingredients:

- 400 Grams Ground Beef
- 2 Tablespoons Ghee
- 4.5 Ounces Goat Cheese
- 1 Yellow Onion, Large & Sliced
- 1 Tablespoon Swerve
- ½ Teaspoon Sea Salt, Fine

Directions:

1. Start by placing your goat cheese in your freezer, leaving it for a half hour.
2. Slice your onion, and then add two tablespoons of ghee into a pan with your onion. Cook for fifteen to twenty minutes, stirring occasionally. Cook until caramelized.
3. Add in your liquid sweetener, cooking for another five minutes. Make sure to stir so that your onions do not burn.
4. Heat your oven to 400, and then remove your cheese from the freezer.
5. Create two patties, and then place a piece of cheese in the middle of each. Cover it so that the cheese doesn't start to ooze out when cooking.
6. Use your ghee to grease an ovenproof skillet, and then add your burgers into it. Season with salt, and cook for seven to eight minutes.
7. Remove from the skillet, and let them cool for five minutes.
8. Top with onions and serve.

Cajun Snow Crab

Serves: 2

Calories: 643

Fat: 51 Grams

Protein: 41 Grams

Fiber: 1 Gram

Net Carbs: 3 Grams

Time: 15 Minutes

Ingredients:

- 1 Lemon, Quartered
- 3 Tablespoons Cajun Seasoning
- 4 Snow Crab Legs, Precooked & Defrosted
- Golden Ghee
- 2 Bay Leaves

Directions:

1. Start by filling a pot with salted water, and place it over high heat. Add in lemon juice, and then toss in your lemon quarters. Add in your Cajun seasoning as well as your bay leaves, boiling for a full minute.
2. Add your crab legs, making sure they're covered by water. Boil for five to eight minutes, and they should stay submerged.
3. Serve with melted ghee for dipping.

Leek & Bacon Frittata

Serves: 2

Calories: 575

Fiber: 1 Gram

Protein: 46 Grams

Fat: 44 Grams

Net Carbs: 3 Grams

Time: 35 Minutes

Ingredients:

- 8 Ounces Bacon, Uncured
- 8 Eggs, Large
- ¼ Cup Leek, Sliced (White Portion Only)
- 1/3 Cup Parmesan Cheese, Grated
- 2 Teaspoons Thyme Leaves, Fresh & Chopped
- 1 Tablespoon Lemon Juice, Fresh
- ½ Cup Heavy Whipping Cream
- ¼ Teaspoon Black Pepper
- ½ Teaspoon Sea Salt, Fine

Directions:

1. Start by heating your oven to 350.
2. Take a ten inch ovenproof cast iron skillet, placing it over medium-high heat. Once it's hot, add in your bacon, cooing until crispy. This will take about three to four minutes on each side, and then set your bacon aside.
3. Add your leeks to the bacon fat left in your pan, sautéing for three minutes.
4. Remove your leeks from the pan, and let it cool. Leave remaining bacon fat in your pan.
5. Beat your eggs in a bowl before whisking your heavy cream, parmesan cheese, thyme, pepper, salt, lemon juice and cooled leek together. Pour this over your skillet, and then add your bacon to the top.
6. Bake your eggs until golden brown, cooking for about eighteen minutes.
7. Let it sit before slicing.

Spiced Lobster Salad

Serves: 1

Calories: 91

Fiber: 0 Grams

Protein: 2 Grams

Fat: 9 Grams

Net Carbs: 2 Grams

Time: 10 Minutes

Ingredients:

- 1/3 Cup Mayonnaise
- 1 Teaspoon Sriracha
- 1 Tablespoon Lemon Juice, Fresh
- 1 ½ Teaspoons Tarragon, Fresh & Minced
- ¼ Cup Celery, Chopped
- 1 Cup Main Lobster Meat, Precooked
- Sea Salt to Taste

Directions:

1. Mix your lemon, sriracha, salt, mayonnaise and tarragon together.
2. Stir in your celery and lobster, mixing well before serving.

Walnut Pork Chops

Serves: 2

Calories: 352

Fiber: 1 Grams

Protein: 47 Grams

Fat: 17 Grams

Net Carbs: 1 Gram

Time: 30 Minutes

Ingredients:

- 3 Tablespoons Walnuts, Crushed
- 2 Pork Chops, Boneless
- 1 Egg, Large
- Sea Salt & Black Pepper
- 3 Tablespoons Parmesan Cheese, Grated

Directions:

1. Start by heating your oven to 400.
2. Place parchment paper on a baking sheet, and then take a shallow dish. Mix the walnuts, salt, pepper and parmesan cheese together.
3. Lightly beat your egg in another shallow dish.
4. Dip your pork chop in the egg, and then dip them in the walnut mixture. Place it on the baking sheet, and cook for ten minutes.
5. Flip and continue baking for another ten minutes. Serve warm.

Easy Black Pepper Chicken

Serves: 2

Calories: 422

Fiber: 2 Grams

Protein: 76 Grams

Fat: 10 Grams

Net Carbs: 4 Grams

Time: 1 Hour 5 Minutes

Ingredients:

- ½ Cup Sake
- ½ Cup Chicken Broth
- 1 Teaspoon Tamari
- 1 Tablespoon Creole Seasoning
- 2 Garlic Cloves, Minced
- 3 Tablespoons Oyster Sauce
- 1 Teaspoon Ground Ginger
- 1 Teaspoon Black Pepper
- 1 Teaspoon Chili Powder
- ½ Red Onion, Sliced
- 1 lb Chicken Tender, Cut into 1 Inch Pieces
- ½ Red Bell Pepper, Cut into Strips

Directions:

1. Whisk your sake, broth, oyster sauce, tamari, garlic, creole seasoning, ginger, pepper and chili powder together.
2. Add your chicken, onion, and red bell pepper, tossing to coat. Let it marinate for thirty minutes in the fridge.
3. Turn your oven to 350.
4. In an ovenproof cast iron skillet, transfer the chicken and remaining marinade to this pan.
5. Bake until cooked through, which will take about twenty-five minutes. During this time you'll need to stir at least twice while baking.

Butter & Herb Scallops

Serves: 4

Calories: 306

Fiber: 0 Grams

Protein: 19 Grams

Fat: 24 Grams

Net Carbs: 4 Grams

Time: 20 Minutes

Ingredients:

- 8 Tablespoons Butter, Divided
- 1 lb Sea Scallops, Cleaned
- Black Pepper to Taste
- 1 Lemon, Juiced
- 2 Teaspoons Garlic, Minced
- 2 Teaspoons Basil, Fresh & Chopped
- 1 Teaspoon Thyme, Fresh & Chopped

Directions:

1. Pat your scallops dry using a paper towel, and then season with black pepper.
2. Cook over medium heat in a skillet, using two tablespoons of butter.
3. Arrange your scallops in the skillet, and sear on each side. They should be golden brown, which will take about two and a half minutes on each side.
4. Remove your scallops from the skillet, setting it aside.
5. Add the rest of your six tablespoons of butter into your skillet, sautéing your garlic for three minutes.
6. Stir in your basil, lemon juice, and thyme. Return your scallops to the skillet, and turn them to coat in the sauce.
7. Serve while warm.

Garlic Shrimp

Serves: 2

Calories: 308

Fiber: 0 Grams

Protein: 43 Grams

Fat: 14 Grams

Net Carbs: 4 Grams

Time: 20 Minutes

Ingredients:

- 2 Garlic Cloves, Minced
- 2 Tablespoons Golden Ghee
- Sea Salt & Pepper to Taste
- 20 Medium Shrimp, Deveined & Peeled
- Red Pepper Flakes to Taste
- 1 Tablespoon Parmesan Cheese, Grated

Directions:

1. Melt your ghee in a skillet over medium-high heat, and then add in your garlic once hot. Cook for one to two minutes, but make sure your garlic doesn't brown.
2. Add in your shrimp, cooing for another two minutes.
3. Add in your salt, pepper and red pepper flakes, sautéing for five minutes. Your shrimp should be cooked all the way through.
4. Add in your parmesan cheese, stirring before serving.

Chicken & Broccoli Alfredo

Serves: 2

Calories: 632

Fiber: 1 Gram

Protein: 58 Grams

Fat: 44 Grams

Net Carbs: 1 Gram

Time: 35 Minutes

Ingredients:

- 1/3 Cup Mascarpone
- 2 Chicken Breasts, Skinless & Boneless
- 1/3 Cup Broccoli Florets
- 2 Teaspoon Garlic, Minced
- ¼ Teaspoon Lemon Pepper Seasoning
- 2 Tablespoons Asiago Cheese, Shaved
- 1 Teaspoon Sea Salt, Fine
- 2 Tablespoons Golden Ghee
- 3 Tablespoons Heavy Whipping Cream

Directions:

1. Fill a large pot with water, and boil over high heat.
2. Add your chicken breasts in, making sure they're fully submerged. Reduce to low heat, simmering while covered for twenty minutes.
3. Remove your chicken before setting your chicken to the side.
4. Steam your broccoli until tender for six minutes.
5. Drain, and then chop your broccoli into small pieces.
6. Heat your mascarpone in a medium skillet, adding in your garlic, salt, ghee, heavy cream, and lemon pepper seasoning. Reduce the heat once the mixture is hot, and then add in your broccoli. Cook for five minutes, making sure to stir frequently.
7. Shred your chicken, discarding tough or fatty bits. Add the shredded chicken to your skillet, cooking for about two minutes.
8. Divide this Alfredo between two places, and then sprinkle with your asiago cheese. Serve.

Pumpkin Curry

Serves: 2

Calories: 540

Fiber: 6 Grams

Protein: 54 Grams

Fat: 32 Grams

Net Carbs: 7 Grams

Time: 25 Minutes

Ingredients:

- 7 Ounces Pumpkin Puree
- ½ Cup Coconut Milk, Unsweetened
- 1 Tablespoon Lime Juice, Fresh
- 1 Teaspoon Curry Powder
- 2 Tablespoons Basil Leaves, Chopped
- 2 Tablespoons Golden Ghee
- ½ White Onion, Small & Chopped
- ½ Teaspoon Ground Coriander
- ½ Teaspoon Ground Ginger
- ½ Teaspoon Ground Cinnamon
- ½ Teaspoon Sea Salt + Additional to Season
- ½ Teaspoon Red Pepper Flakes
- 1 lb Chicken Tenders
- Black Pepper to taste
- 2 Tablespoons Olive Oil

Directions:

1. Take your pumpkin puree, coconut milk, lime juice, basil, curry powder, ghee, coriander, cinnamon, salt, red pepper flakes and ginger. Blend together in a blender, pouring into a saucepan after blended. Turn the heat to medium.
2. Heat your olive oil over medium heat in another skillet, and then season your chicken tenders with salt and pepper. Once your oil is hot, cook on each side for three minutes.

3. Cut your chicken into one inch pieces, and then add them to your pumpkin curry.
4. Turn your heat to low, cooking for another five to ten minutes.
5. Serve warm.

Chapter 9: Side Dishes

With some of the main dinner entrees above, you'll need side dishes. Here are some keto friendly and tasty side dishes for you to try!

Kale Slaw

Serves: 6

Calories: 147

Fiber: 2.5 Grams

Protein: 3.4 Grams

Fat: 13.3 Grams

Net Carbs: 3.5 Grams

Time: 10 Minutes

Ingredients:

- 1 Bunch Kale
- 2 ½ Cups Red Cabbage, shredded
- ½ Cup Carrot, Grated
- 1 ¼ Cup Green Cabbage, Shredded
- Salt & Pepper to taste
- 1 Tablespoon Lemon Juice, Fresh
- 1/3 Cup Mayonnaise
- ¼ Cup Pumpkin Seeds

Directions:

1. Slice your cabbage and kale thin. Make sure your cabbage is grated, and add everything together.
2. Serve with mayonnaise and lemon juice.

Roasted Broccoli

Serves: 4

Calories: 179

Fiber: 3.9 Grams

Protein: 4.3 Grams

Fat: 14.3 Grams

Net Carbs: 6.9 Grams

Time: 15 Minutes

Ingredients:

- 2 Broccoli, Medium
- 2 Tablespoons Lemon Juice, Fresh
- 2 Cloves Garlic, Minced
- ¼ Cup Ghee, Melted
- Salt & Pepper to Taste

Directions:

1. Start by heating your oven to 450, and then wash and cut your broccoli.
2. Mix in your garlic and your melted ghee.
3. Place the broccoli in a baking dish, tossing to combine, and then squeeze the lemon juice over it before seasoning with salt and pepper.
4. Bake for twelve to fifteen minutes.
5. Allow to cool before serving.

Creamy Spinach

Serves: 4

Calories: 195

Fiber: 2 Grams

Protein: 3 Grams

Fat: 20 Grams

Net Carbs: 1 Gram

Time: 40 Minutes

Ingredients:

- 1 Tablespoon Butter
- Nutmeg, Salt & Pepper to Taste
- ¾ Cup Heavy Whipping Cream
- ¼ Cup Herbed Chicken Stock
- 4 Cups Spinach, Stemmed & Washed
- ½ Sweet Onion, Sliced Thin

Directions:

1. Add butter to a large skillet putting it over medium heat.
2. Sauté your onion for about five minutes. It should caramelize lightly.
3. Stir in your chicken stock, heavy cream, nutmeg, salt, pepper and spinach.
4. Sauté for another five minutes. Your spinach should become wilted. Continue to cook until tender, and your sauce should thicken.
5. This will take about fifteen minutes, and you'll want to serve immediately.

Crisp Zucchini

Serves: 4

Calories: 94

Fiber: 0 Grams

Protein: 4 Grams

Fat: 8 Grams

Net Carbs: 1 Gram

Time: 25 Minutes

Ingredients:

- 2 Tablespoons Butter
- ½ Cup Parmesan Cheese, Grated
- Salt & Pepper to Taste
- 4 Zucchini, Cut Into Round (1/4 Inch Thick)

Directions:

1. Place your butter in a skillet. Turn the heat to medium-high.
2. Sauté your zucchini until tender. It should take five minutes before lightly browned.
3. Spread the zucchini in the skillet before sprinkling your parmesan over it.
4. Do not stir, and cook until melted. This should take about five minutes.
5. Serve immediately.

Cauliflower Mash

Serves: 6

Calories: 225

Fiber: 3.1 Grams

Protein: 5.6 Grams

Fat: 20.8 Grams

Net Carbs: 7.3 Grams

Time: 20 Minutes

Ingredients:

- 1 Cauliflower, Large
- 1 Celeriac, Small
- ¼ Cup Ghee
- Salt & Pepper to Taste
- 1 Tablespoon Rosemary, Chopped
- 1 Cup Cream Cheese, Full Fat
- 1 Tablespoon Thyme, Chopped

Directions:

1. Start by dicing and peeling your celeriac. The pieces should be about one inch. The cauliflower will need chopped into small florets as well. Chop your rosemary and thyme if needed.
2. Take a large pan and heat the ghee over it using medium-high heat. Add in your chopped herbs, cooing until fragrant.
3. Add your celeriac and cauliflower before seasoning with salt and pepper.
4. Cook for five minutes, stirring to prevent burning.
5. Lower your heat and then cover, cooing for twelve to fifteen minutes. It should become soft.
6. Place it in a blender, pulsing until smooth.
7. Add in your cream cheese and continue to pulse.
8. Top with butter after transferring to a serving bowl.

Easy Brussel Sprouts

Serves: 4

Calories: 179

Fiber: 4.8 Grams

Protein: 4.2 Grams

Fat: 14.1 Grams

Net Carbs: 6.8 Grams

Time: 40 Minutes

Ingredients:

- 1.1 lbs Brussel Sprouts
- ½ Lemon, Juiced
- ¼ Cup Ghee, Melted
- ½ Teaspoon Sea Salt, Fine
- ¼ Teaspoon Pepper
- ¼ Cup Pine Nuts, Toasted

Directions:

1. Start by turning your oven to 400, and then halve your Brussel sprouts. If they're too big, you'll want to quarter them.
2. Pour your melted ghee over them.
3. Drizzle your lemon juice on top, and then season using salt and pepper.
4. Place in a baking dish, baking for 25-35 minutes. Cook until tender.
5. Toss in your toasted pine nuts before serving.

Ranch Broccoli Bites

Serves: 4

Calories: 312

Fiber: 2 Grams

Protein: 18 Grams

Fat: 26 Grams

Net Carbs: 4 Grams

Time: 1 Hour

Ingredients:

- ¾ Cup Sour Cream, Full Fat
- 8 Ounces Bacon, Uncured
- 4 Cups Broccoli Florets
- 2 Tablespoons Mayonnaise
- 1 Cup Cheddar Cheese, Shredded
- 2 Tablespoons Tangy Ranch Rub

Directions:

1. Start by heating your oven to 400.
2. Bake your bacon on a baking tray until crispy.
3. Mix your mayonnaise, sour cream and tangy ranch rub together in a bowl.
4. Put your broccoli in a dish, and then pour the sour cream mixture over it. Top with cheese, baking for a half hour.
5. Crumble your bacon over it before serving.

Green Beans

Serves: 4

Calories: 104

Fiber: 1 Gram

Protein: 4 Grams

Fat: 9 Grams

Net Carbs: 1 Gram

Time: 20 Minutes

Ingredients:

- 1 lb Green Beans, Stemmed
- ¼ Cup Parmesan Cheese, Grated
- Sea Salt & Pepper to Taste
- 1 Teaspoon Garlic, Minced
- 2 Tablespoons Olive Oil

Directions:

1. Start by heating your oven to 425. Line your baking sheet before setting it aside.
2. Toss your green beans, olive oils and garlic together in a bowl.
3. Season your green beans using salt and pepper, and then spread them on the roasted pan. Cook for ten minutes, stirring once in the middle of it.
4. Top with parmesan before serving.

Southern Green Beans

Serves: 4

Calories: 93

Fiber: 4 Grams

Protein: 2 Grams

Fat: 8 Grams

Net Carbs: 4 Grams

Time: 15 Minutes

Ingredients:

- 4 Cups Green Beans, Trimmed
- 2 Tablespoons Golden Ghee
- 2 Garlic Cloves, Minced
- Sea Salt & Red Pepper to Taste

Directions:

1. Salt a pot of water, bringing it to a boil.
2. Add in your green beans, cooking for three minutes.
3. Drain them and plunge them into a bowl of ice water.
4. Once cooled, drain them and set them to the side.
5. Melt your ghee over medium heat, and then add your garlic, red pepper flakes and salt until softened. It should take about a minute.
6. Add in your green beans, and then coo for three minutes.
7. Serve warm.

Asparagus & Walnuts

Serves: 4

Calories: 124

Fiber: 2 Grams

Protein: 3 Grams

Fat: 12 Grams

Net Carbs: 2 Grams

Time: 15 Minutes

Ingredients:

- ¾ lb Asparagus, Trimmed
- ¼ Cup Walnuts, Chopped
- Sea Salt & Pepper
- 1 ½ Tablespoons Olive Oil

Directions:

1. Take a large skillet and add your oil, turning it over medium-high heat.
2. Sauté for five minutes. Your spears should be tender and browned lightly.
3. Season with salt and pepper, and then remove from heat.
4. Toss in your walnuts before serving.

Rosti

Serves: 8

Calories: 171

Fiber: 0 Grams

Protein: 5 Grams

Fat: 14 Grams

Net Carbs: 3 Grams

Time: 30 Minutes

Ingredients:

- 1 Cup Acorn Squash, Shredded
- 2 Teaspoons Garlic, Minced
- 1 Cup Celeriac, Shredded
- 2 Tablespoons Parmesan Cheese, Grated
- 1 Teaspoon Thyme, Chopped
- 2 Tablespoons Butter
- 8 Bacon Slices, Chopped
- Sea Salt & Pepper to Taste

Directions:

1. Coo your bacon for about five minutes. It should be crispy.
2. Let it cool, and then in a bowl mix your celeriac, parmesan, garlic, squash and thyme together. Season generously with salt and pepper before putting this bowl to the side.
3. Remove your bacon, and stir it into the bowl.
4. Reserve tow tablespoons of bacon fat and then get rid of the rest.
5. Put the bacon fat and butter in the skillet, and reduce the heat to medium-low.
6. Transfer your squash mixture to the skillet, and then cook. Let it form a round patty about an inch thick. The bottom should be grips and golden. This will take about five minutes.
7. Flip and cook for another five minutes. Take off of heat.
8. Cut into eight pieces before serving.

122

Chapter 10: Keto Desserts

If you'd like to skip a snack after breakfast or lunch, you can sometimes squeeze in a keto dessert. Otherwise, these can be used for snacks as well.

Keto Whipped Cream

This is for toppings, and is not a dessert on its own. However, you should only use it on recipes that call for it.

Serves: 6

Calories: 69

Fiber: 0 Grams

Protein: 0 Grams

Fat: 7 Grams

Net Carbs: 1 Gram

Time: 30 Seconds

Ingredients:

- 1 Cup Heavy Whipping Cream
- 1 Tablespoon Vanilla Bean Sweetener (Next Recipe)

Directions:

1. Blend in a blender until it turns into a fluffy cream. This will take ten to fifteen seconds. Its best if served immediately, but you can keep it in the fridge for a day.

Keto Vanilla Bean Sweetener

This will be used in different recipes, but is not to be eaten on its own.

Yields: 1 Cup

Calories: 0

Fiber: 0 Grams

Protein: 0 Grams

Fat: 0 Grams

Net Carbs: 2 Grams

Time: 15 Minutes

Ingredients:

- 1 Drop Liquid Sweetener
- ½ Cup Erythritol
- 2 Teaspoon Vanilla Bean Extract, Pure
- 1 Cup Water
- 1 Vanilla Bean Pod, Halved Lengthwise & Deseeded

Directions:

1. Bring your water to a boil, and then reduce to low. Add in your vanilla extract, Erythritol, liquid sweetener, and vanilla seeds.
2. Simmer, stirring frequently. It should reduce by half, which will take about ten minutes.
3. Pour into a tight fitting jar, and it'll keep for about two weeks in the fridge.

Black Forest Pudding

Serves: 4

Calories: 166

Fiber: 4 Grams

Protein: 4 Grams

Fat: 16 Grams

Net Carbs: 4 Grams

Time: 30 Minutes

Ingredients:

- 1 Cup Almond Milk, Unsweetened
- 1 Cup Heavy Whipping Cream
- 3 Cherries, Pitted & Chopped
- 2 Egg Yolks, Large
- Sea Salt to Taste
- ½ Cup Cocoa Powder, Unsweetened
- ¼ Cup Vanilla Bean Sweetener

Directions:

1. Take a medium pan, and heat your almond milk, cocoa powder, cherries, heavy cream and salt together. Coo over heat for three minutes, and then remove the cherries using a slotted spoon. Set the cherries aside.
2. Take a bowl and beat your egg yolks, and slowly pour in your hot cream mixture as you whisk continuously.
3. Pour this mixture back into the pot, cooking for another fifteen minutes. Make sure to stir constantly and scrape the sides and bottom. It should thicken, and then you'll need to add in the sweetener.
4. Pour your mix in an airtight container, and refrigerate for about two hours.
5. Transfer to an ice cream maker, following manufacturer's instructions.
6. Fold in your cherries once the ice cream is ready, and then allow to firm for three hours.

Sage & Blackberry Ice Pops

Serves: 6-8

Calories: 10

Fiber: 1 Gram

Protein: 0 Grams

Fat: 0 Grams

Net Carbs: 1 Gram

Time: 5 Minutes

Ingredients:

- ½ Cup Water
- 1 Cup Blackberries
- 2 Sage Leaves, Fresh
- 1 Teaspoon Vanilla Bean Sweetener

Directions:

1. Blend until smooth, and then place in ice pop sleeves.
2. Freeze overnight.

Strawberries & Cream Cake

Serves: 1

Calories: 719

Fiber: 4 Grams

Protein: 15 Grams

Fat: 67 Grams

Net Carbs: 6 Grams

Time: 15 Minutes

Ingredients:

- ¼ Cup Vanilla Bean Sweetener
- 2 Eggs, Large
- 2 Tablespoons Golden Ghee
- ¼ Cup Almond Flour
- 2 Tablespoons Cream Cheese, Room Temperature
- ¼ Cup Whipped Cream
- 4 Strawberries, Hulled & Chopped into Hunks

Directions:

1. Blend your eggs, sweetener, cream cheese and ghee together. Scrap into a microwave safe mug.
2. Stir in your strawberries and almond flower.
3. Microwave for four minutes, and let cool before topping with whipped cream to serve.

Cinnamon Mug Cake

Serves: 1

Calories: 333

Fiber: 4.4 Grams

Protein: 11.8 Grams

Fat: 15.7 Grams

Protein: 11.8 Grams

Net Carbs: 3.9 Grams

Time: 10 Minutes

Ingredients:

- 2 Tablespoons Almond Flour
- 1 Tablespoon Coconut Flour
- 1 Tablespoon Swerve
- 1 Egg, Large
- 1 Tablespoon Melted Butter
- 1/8 Teaspoon Baking Soda
- ½ Teaspoon Cinnamon

Directions

1. Combine all your dry ingredients in a mug, mixing well.
2. Add in your butter and egg, mixing well.
3. Microwave for 70-90 seconds, and then top with whipped cream if desired.

Sage & Berry Fruit Salad

Serves: 1

Calories: 81

Fiber: 9 Grams

Protein: 2 Grams

Fat: 1 Gram

Net Carbs: 9 Grams

Time: 5 Minutes

Ingredients:

- ½ Cup Raspberries
- ¼ Cup Strawberries, Sliced
- ½ Cup Blackberries
- 1 Teaspoon Lemon Juice, Fresh
- 1 Sage Leaf, Fresh & Chopped
- 1 Tablespoon Blueberries
- 1 Teaspoon Vanilla Bean Sweetener

Directions:

1. Toss together before serving.

Orange Creamsicle Fat Bomb

Yields: 12

Calories: 178

Fiber: 0 Grams

Protein: 1.04 Grams

Fat: 19 Grams

Net Carbs: 0.95 Grams

Time: 3 Hours 10 Minutes

Ingredients:

- 10 Drops Liquid Stevia
- 1 Teaspoon Orange Vanilla Mio
- 4 Ounces Cream Cheese, Room Temperature
- ½ Cup Coconut Oil
- ½ Cup Heavy Whipping Cream

Directions:

1. Blend all ingredients together, and then spread into a silicone tray, freezing for two to three hours.

Lime & Strawberry Sorbet

Serves: 6

Calories: 104

Fiber: 1 Gram

Protein: 5 Grams

Fat: 8 Grams

Net Carbs: 4 Grams

Time: 5 Minutes

Ingredients:

- 3 Cups Strawberries, Chopped
- 1 Cup Heavy Whipping Cream
- Zest of 1 Lime
- 2 Tablespoons Vanilla Bean Sweetener
- 3 Tablespoons Gelatin

Directions:

1. Blend your strawberries, lime zest, gelatin, and heavy cream together in a blender. Add in your sweetener, and blend for another thirty seconds.
2. Pour mixture into an ice cream maker and follow the instructions of your marker to make sorbet.
3. Let it freeze for a minimum of two hours.

Orange Maple Spiced Mug Cake

Serves: 1

Calories: 392

Fiber: 2 Grams

Proteins: 67 Grams

Fat: 37 Grams

Net Carbs: 2 Grams

Time: 15 Minutes

Ingredients:

- 2 Tablespoons Almond Flour
- ½ Teaspoon Maple Extract
- ½ Teaspoon Orange Extract
- 1 Egg, Large
- 2 Tablespoons Vanilla Bean Sweetener
- ½ Teaspoon Baking Powder
- 2 Tablespoons Golden Ghee
- 1/8 Teaspoon Ground Cinnamon

Directions:

1. Crack your egg into a mug that's microwave safe, and beat lightly with a fork. Add in your sweetener, and then add in your orange and maple extract. Make sure to stir well.
2. Mix your baking powder, almond flour, and cinnamon in a bowl before adding the mix into your mug.
3. Stir in your ghee, and then microwave for two minutes on high.
4. Let it cool before eating. You do not need to remove it from the mug.

Chapter 11: Keto Home Staples

There are some foods that people have a hard time giving up. For example, you may find it hard to give up crackers. That's what this recipe is all about.

Keto Nutella

Serves: 2

Calories: 193

Fiber: 2.9 Grams

Protein: 3.9 Grams

Fat: 18.7 Grams

Net Carbs: 3 Grams

Time: 30 Minutes

Ingredients:

- 1 Cup Hazelnuts, Peeled
- ½ Cup Almonds
- 1 Cup Macadamia Nuts
- 3.5 Ounces Dark Chocolate
- ½ Teaspoon Vanilla Powder
- 1 Tablespoon Cocoa Powder
- 2 Tablespoons Powdered Swerve
- 1 Tablespoon Virgin Coconut Oil

Directions:

1. Start by heating your oven to 375.
2. Spread your macadamia nuts, hazelnuts, and almonds on a baking tray. Bake for eight to ten minutes, making sure they're lightly browned.
3. Let them cool for fifteen minutes after removing them from the oven.
4. Melt your coconut oil and chocolate over a double boiler, stirring while melting.
5. Use a food processor, pulsing the nuts until you get a smooth texture.
6. Add in your coconut oil, melted chocolate, cacao powder, vanilla powder and powdered swerve.

7. Blend until smooth, and store in the fridge for three months.

Keto Bread

Yields: 1 Loaf (14 Slices)

Calories: 213

Fiber: 0.3 Grams

Protein: 14.7 Grams

Fat: 18.1 Grams

Net Carbs: 1.3 Grams

Time: 1 Hour 15 Minutes

Ingredients:

- ¼ Cup Butter, Melted
- 1 ½ Cup Cream Cheese, Full Fat & Room Temperature
- ¼ Cup Heavy Whipping Cream
- ¼ Cup Extra Virgin Olive Oil
- 4 Eggs, Large
- 2 Teaspoons Cream of Tartar
- 1 Teaspoon Glucomanna Powder
- 1 Teaspoon Baking Soda
- 1 2/3 Cup Whey Protein, Unflavored
- ½ Teaspoon Sea Salt, Fine

Directions:

1. Turn your oven to 325. Place your salt and cream cheese in a bowl, whisking together.
2. Add in your olive oil and melted ghee.
3. Add in your eggs and heavy whipping cream, beating until combined.
4. Sift your baking soda, cream of tartar and glucomanna powder into the batter. Stir often.
5. Sift in your protein powder, whisking to avoid clumps.
6. Pour into a loaf pan, and then bake for fifty minutes.
7. Let cool for ten to fifteen minutes before slicing.

Keto Honey

Yields: ¾ Cup

Serving: 1 Tablespoon

Calories: 31

Fiber: 11.9 Grams

Protein: 0.5 Grams

Fat: 0.1 Grams

Net Carbs: 1.6 Grams

Ingredients:

- 1-2 Tablespoons Water, Warm
- ½ Cup Sukrin Syrup, Clear
- 2 Tablespoons Bee Pollen

Directions:

1. Blend your bee pollen with a tablespoon of warm water. Let it sit for five to ten minutes, and then pulse until it gets creamy. If you need to add the other tablespoon of water do so before adding your sukrin syrup.
2. Pulse until your syrup is dissolved.
3. Keep in an airtight jar at room temperature.

Coconut Butter

Yields: 1 ¼ Cup

Serving: 2 Tablespoons

Calories: 180

Fiber: 4.8 Grams

Protein: 1.9 Grams

Fat: 17.6 Grams

Net Carbs: 1.9 Grams

Time: 10 Minutes

Ingredients:

- 4 Cups Shredded Coconut, Unsweetened
- ¼ Teaspoon Sea Salt, Fine

Directions:

1. Place your coconut in a food processor, processing until it reaches the desired consistency. You'll need to process for about eight minutes.
2. Add in your salt, and then process again to distribute.

Savory Pie Crust

Yield: 1 Pie Crust (8 Slices)

Serving: 1 Slice

Calories: 177

Fiber: 2.5 Grams

Protein: 13.2 Grams

Fat: 11 Grams

Net Carbs: 1.3 Grams

Time: 30 Minutes

Ingredients:

- 2 Cups Pork Rinds
- 1 Cup Almond Flour
- ¼ Cup Flax meal
- ½ Teaspoon Sea Salt, Fine
- 2 Eggs, Large

Directions:

1. Turn your oven to 400.
2. Blend your pork rinds to make a powder. Remove any skin bits if they are left.
3. Place the powdered pork rinds in a bowl, adding in your flax meal and almond flour. Add salt if you feel it's needed.
4. Crack in your eggs, mixing well until it forms a dough. Place into a pie pan, and then bake in the oven for twelve to fifteen minutes.

Sweet Pie Crust

Yields: 1 Pie Crust (8 Slices)

Calories: 179

Fiber: 2.2 Grams

Protein: 8.4 Grams

Fat: 15.5 Grams

Net Carbs: 2.3 Grams

Time: 25 Minutes

Ingredients:

- 1 ¾ Cup Almond Flour
- ¼ Cup Swerve, Powdered
- 1 Egg, Large
- 2 Tablespoons Extra Virgin Coconut Oil
- ¼ Cup Vanilla Whey Protein

Directions:

1. Turn your oven to 350.
2. Mix all dry ingredients together, and then add in your coconut oil and egg. Mix together thoroughly.
3. Place the dough in a pan, and then bake for twelve to fifteen minutes.

Tortillas

Yields: 10 Tortillas

Serving Size: 1 Tortilla

Calories: 165

Fiber: 5.7 Grams

Protein: 5.1 Grams

Fat: 14 Grams

Net Carbs: 1.5 Grams

Time: 1 Hour

Ingredients:

- 1 Cup Almond Flour
- ¾ Cup Flax meal
- 1 Teaspoon Sea Salt, Fine
- 2 Tablespoons Chia Seeds, Grounded
- 2 Tablespoon Psyllium Husks, Whole
- ¼ Cup Coconut Flour
- 2 Tablespoons Coconut Oil
- 1 Cup Water, Lukewarm

Directions:

1. Mix your psyllium husks, almond flour, coconut flour and flax meal together.
2. Add your ground chia seeds, and then blend everything to a powder in your blender.
3. Pour in your water, combining well with your hands to make a dough. Add more water if necessary.
4. Refrigerate for up to an hour, and then cut the dough into pieces.
5. Roll out, and then cut into circles to make ten tortillas. With any leftover dough, you can cook it longer to make nacho chips.
6. Use ghee to grease a pan, and then cook one to two minutes on each side.

Onion & Rosemary Crackers

Yields: 11-12 Crackers

Serves: 3-4

Calories: 103

Fiber: 2.8 Grams

Protein: 3.6 Grams

Fat: 8.9 Grams

Net Carbs: 1 Gram

Time: 25 Minutes

Ingredients:

- 2 Tablespoons Rosemary, Chopped
- ½ Teaspoon Onion Powder
- 1 Cup Almonds, Ground
- ½ Cup Flax Seeds
- 1 Teaspoon Baking Soda
- ½ Teaspoon Pepper
- ½ Teaspoon Sea Salt, Fine
- 1 Egg, Large
- 1 Tablespoon Olive Oil

Directions:

1. Start by heating your oven to 340.
2. Process your flaxseeds and rosemary in a food processor to make a fine blend.
3. Add in your ground almonds, onion, baking soda, salt and pepper, mixing well.
4. Transfer to a bowl and then add in your egg. Whisk in, and then add in your olive oil.
5. Add your dry ingredients to your wet ingredients, rolling it into a ball of dough.
6. Roll out to a one quarter inch thickness.
7. Use a biscuit cutter to cut into cracker shapes, and then bake for twelve to fifteen minutes. They should be golden brown.

Ketchup

Yields: 2 Cups

Serving Size: 1 Tablespoon

Calories: 4.8

Fiber: 0.23 Grams

Protein: 0.18 Grams

Fat: 0.03 Grams

Net Carbs: 0.84 Grams

Time: 15 Minutes

Ingredients:

- 1 Small Onion
- 2 Cloves Garlic
- 1/8 Teaspoon Cloves, Ground
- 1/8 Teaspoon Allspice, Ground
- 1 Cup Tomato Puree
- ¼ Cup Apple Cider Vinegar
- 3-6 Drops Stevia
- 2 Tablespoons Swerve
- 1 Teaspoon Sea Salt, Fine
- ½ Teaspoon Black Pepper
- ¼ Cup Water

Directions:

1. Peel your onion before cutting. Cut your garlic into small pieces as well.
2. Place all ingredients into a pan, simmering over low heat for five to ten minutes. You'll need to add more water if it becomes too thick.
3. Place the mix in a blender, blending until smooth.
4. It'll keep in the fridge for up to a month.

Mayonnaise

Yields: 1 Cup

Serving Size: 1 Tablespoon

Calories: 111

Fiber: 0 Grams

Protein: 0.17 Grams

Fat: 12.5 Grams

Net Carbs: 0.1 Grams

Time: 10 Minutes

Ingredients:

- ¾ Cup Avocado Oil
- 1 Egg Yolk, Large
- 1 Teaspoon Dijon Mustard
- 1 Tablespoon Apple Cider Vinegar
- 1 Tablespoon Lemon Juice, Fresh
- ¼ Teaspoon Sea Salt, Fine

Directions:

1. All of your ingredients should be room temperature before you start.
2. Separate your egg white from your egg yolk, and then mix your Dijon mustard with your egg yolk in a bowl. Make sure it's mixed well.
3. Whisk to blend, and then slowly add in your oil.
4. Keep pouring until it looks like mayonnaise, and then continue to mix well.
5. Add in your vinegar, salt and lemon juice, whisking well.

Caesar Dressing

Yields: 1 ½ Cups

Calories: 180

Fiber: 0 Grams

Protein: 1 Gram

Fat: 20 Grams

Net Carbs: 1 Gram

Time: 15 Minutes

Ingredients:

- 4 Egg Yolks, Large
- Salt & Pepper to Taste
- ¼ Cup Lemon Juice, Fresh
- Dash Worcestershire Sauce
- 1 Cup Olive Oil
- ¼ Cup Wine Vinegar
- 2 Teaspoons Garlic, Minced
- ½ Teaspoon Dry Mustard

Directions:

1. Add your egg yolks, vinegar, garlic, Worcestershire, and mustard to a pan, placing it over low heat.
2. Whisk constantly as you cook for about five minutes. The sauce should thicken, and it'll bubble lightly.
3. Remove from heat, and let it cool for ten minutes.
4. Place in a bowl, whisking in your olive oil.
5. Whisk in your lemon juice, seasoning with salt and pepper to taste. This will keep for three days in the fridge.

Chapter 12: Keto Diet Tips

The keto diet is a lifestyle choice, and it can be hard to transition to and stick with. That's why it's important that you follow the meal plan for the first two weeks, and it'll help you to get used to everything. In this chapter you'll find a few more tips that can help your keto diet to be a success.

Tip #1 Give It a Month

It can take two to three weeks to get over the keto flu, and that's only if you do it right on the first time. If you still don't feel good after a month and have made sure that you are doing it right, then it may not be right for you. It's good to set a goal of three to four weeks at least to make sure that you stick with it for long enough that it really starts to work for you. You may not notice great weight loss until you get over this hill.

Tip #2 Hydrate

A lot of people underestimate hydration, especially when they live a busy day to day life. If you stay hydrated, you're less likely to get sick. You're more likely to get over the keto flu a lot faster too. It can be hard to hydrate effectively at first, but as you get into the habit it'll become easier. Hydrating properly will help you to lose weight as well.

Tip #3 Take Probiotics

It's important to have proper bowel movements when you're on the keto diet, especially since the keto flu can cause diarrhea or constipation. Before you go on the keto diet you'll want to make sure you're regular, and you'll want to start taking probiotics to help as soon as you start your diet. It can also be important to pay attention to your fiber intake to make sure everything goes smoothly. This will help you to lose weight faster, exercise easier, and it'll help you to get over the keto flu faster too. It can even help some people avoid the keto flu entirely.

Tip #4 Moderate Protein

It's important that you don't eat too much protein. You may even come out of ketosis if you're eating more protein than your body can handle. This book teaches a standard keto diet, which is not for athletes or weight lifters. Too much protein can change the way your body reacts to ketosis or even if it enters it at all. It's especially important that you keep to a moderate amount of protein if you're only doing a moderate amount of exercise.

Tip #5 Moderate Stress

It's important that you keep your stress down because if you're stressed it can shut down ketosis. Stress will produce stress hormones, which will elevate your blood sugar. This isn't good for prolonged periods of time because it lowers ketones while driving up blood sugar. If you're at a tough time in your life, it's important to reduce stress or start your keto diet later so that you have no issue going into ketosis.

Tip #6 Get Good Sleep

You're not going to be able to function properly if you aren't getting enough sleep. Poor sleep can also affect the way you lose weight. It can also help if you sleep in a room that's completely dark. Remember that lights can decrease your melatonin, which means your body won't be functioning as properly as it should. It can also help you to sleep if you keep your room at a cool temperature.

Chapter 13: Tips for Eating Out

In our day and age it can be almost impossible not to eat out, and if you're on the keto diet that can be difficult. Though, you won't need to give up eating out completely. In this chapter you'll find some tips to help you get the same experience while sticking to your diet.

For Breakfast

This will be one of your most difficult times to try and eat out because most breakfast items aren't naturally keto friendly. You'll need to skip the waffles, pancakes, bagels, and even French toast. You'll want to opt for an omelet or just a few eggs with ham, sausage, steak or bacon on the side. You'll need to skip any toast or hash browns too. Remember that potatoes aren't keto friendly either!

For Lunch

If you're trying to eat out around lunch time the best thing would be a salad with lots of meat. Cobb, garden salad, or Caesar salad is usually a good choice. You'll want to use plenty of olive oil too. Luckily the fiber from the salad should help you to feel full enough that you aren't too hungry before dinner.

For Dinner

The most common thing to order with friends is a burger and fries, but you won't be able to eat that burger bun or those fries. Try to ask if you can get your burger wrapped in lettuce. If they can't, you can just as that no bun is brought out. If they bring a bun out, then take the patty off. You'll need to skip the ketchup too since it's full of sugar. You can use mayonnaise, mustard, sriracha, or even red pepper sauce.

It'd be harder if you're at an Italian restaurant because you'll need to skip the pizza or pasta. You'll want a protein based dinner. Try to request salad or low carb alternatives instead of a carb heavy side too. When ordering Mexican, try to get your ingredients in a bowl instead of a tortilla or burrito rap. You'll need to skip the beans and rice too, so try to add in extra guacamole or sour cream instead.

For Sides

Sides can be difficult because old time favorites such as fries, mashed potatoes, and baked potatoes, corn on the cob, beans, rice, and even banana bread are a no go. You'll want to stick with green beans, broccoli, asparagus, salad or other low carb vegetables.

For Alcohol & Drinks

Don't get juice or soda. You'll want to stick to coffee, tea or water. You can use heavy cream or even half and half instead of milk. Alcohol is something you'll want to avoid mostly too. You'll slow down any fat burning possibilities with too much alcohol, making it impossible to meet your goal. If you do order alcohol, try to avoid cocktails since they have a lot of sugar. Low carb beers can be a good choice, and pure spirits are a good choice too.

Conclusion

Now you have everything that you need to start your keto diet! With the two week meal plan you can get started, but feel free to look at the other recipes or even create your own. You should try to limit yor net carbs to twenty net carbs per day if you want the keto diet to help you lose weight, and you can use many keto calculators online if you're trying to create your own recipe. The ketogenic diet is a lifestyle choice, and it can lead to weight loss and a general happier, healthier you.

Free Bonus!! FREE Keto Recipes, Diet Tips, and much more! Visit the website at: http://KetoDiet.coach to sign up for our newsletter free!

CPSIA information can be obtained
at www.ICGtesting.com
Printed in the USA
BVHW011933150620
581609BV00014B/264

9 781979 505789